DASH DIET

Dash Diet Meal Plan to Lose Weight and Lower Your Blood Pressure

(Delicious Dash Diet Recipes and Menu Plans)

George Chavez

Published by Alex Howard

© **George Chavez**

All Rights Reserved

Dash Diet: Dash Diet Meal Plan to Lose Weight and Lower Your Blood Pressure (Delicious Dash Diet Recipes and Menu Plans)

ISBN 978-1-990169-01-4

All rights reserved. No part of this guide may be reproduced in any form without permission in writing from the publisher except in the case of brief quotations embodied in critical articles or reviews.

Legal & Disclaimer

The information contained in this book is not designed to replace or take the place of any form of medicine or professional medical advice. The information in this book has been provided for educational and entertainment purposes only.

The information contained in this book has been compiled from sources deemed reliable, and it is accurate to the best of the Author's knowledge; however, the Author cannot guarantee its accuracy and validity and cannot be held liable for any errors or omissions. Changes are periodically made to this book. You must consult your doctor or get professional medical advice before using any of the suggested remedies, techniques, or information in this book.

Table of contents

PART 1 1

INTRODUCTION 2

CHAPTER 1: THE FUNDAMENTALS OF DASH DIET 4

What Is The Dash Diet? 4
Fantastic Dash Diet Health Benefits! 5
The Two Types Of Dash 8
Entering The Dash 9
How To Kickstart Your Dash Diet 9
The Serving Chart 10
The Food Groups For Dash 15
Good Salt Alternatives To Know About 16
Awesome Tips For The Journey 17

CHAPTER 2: SAMPLE 7 DAYS MEAL PLAN 19

CHAPTER 3: BREAKFAST RECIPES 21

Simple Blueberry Oatmeal 21
The "Dashing" Chia Pudding 23
The Slow Cooker Chicken Omelet 25
Tasty Spinach Pie 27
Mesmerizing Carrot And Pineapple Mix 29

CHAPTER 4: VEGAN AND VEGETARIAN RECIPES 31

Traditional Black Bean Chili 31
Amazing Broccoli And Cauliflower Soup 33
Mesmerizing Lentil Soup 35
Very Wild Mushroom Pilaf 37
Spicy Cabbage Dish 39

CHAPTER 5: SIDE DISH RECIPES 41

Enjoyable Spinach And Bean Medley 41
Edible Okra Mints 43

TANTALIZING CAULIFLOWER AND DILL MASH 45
SECRET ASIAN GREEN BEANS 47
EXCELLENT ACORN MIX 48

CHAPTER 6: SNACKS RECIPES 49

ELEGANT CORN SALAD 49
QUICK ASPARAGUS BITE 51
AUSPICIOUS ITALIAN SHRIMP SALAD 53
RICKETY NUT MIX 55
SIMPLE FISH STICKS 56

CHAPTER 7: POULTRY RECIPES 58

HEARTY CHICKEN AND VEGGIES 58
ALL-TIME FAVORITE PULLED CHICKEN 60
COOL MEDITERRANEAN CHICKEN 62
SLOW COOKER MEXICAN CHICKEN 64
SWEET POTATO TURKEY BREAST 65

CHAPTER 8: MEAT RECIPES 67

HEALTHY AND JUICY PORK ROAST 67
AUTHENTIC GREEK PORK 69
FOREIGN MOROCCAN LAMB DISH 71
MAPLE PORK TENDERLOIN 73
JUICY HUNGARIAN GOULASH 75

CHAPTER 9: DESSERT RECIPES 77

HEARTY PINEAPPLE PUDDING 77
CRUNCHY ALMOND CHOCOLATE BARS 79
HEALTHY BERRY COBBLER 81
TASTY POACHED APPLES 83
HEART WARMING CINNAMON RICE PUDDING 84

CHAPTER 10: FISH RECIPES 85

HERBED UP SALMON 85
THE ASIAN SALMON DELIGHT 87
THE LEMON AND SPINACH "TROUT" DISH 88
SIMPLE SLOW COOKER TUNA 90

CONCLUSION	92
PATR 2	93
INTRODUCTION	94
WHAT IS DASH DIET?	95
BASIC RULES & BENEFITS OF DASH DIET	97
BREAKFAST RECIPES	101
VERY BERRY MUESLI	101
VEGGIE QUICHE MUFFINS	102
TURKEY SAUSAGE AND MUSHROOM STRATA	103
SUMMER BREAKFAST QUINOA BOWLS	105
STRAWBERRY BREAKFAST SANDWICH	105
STEEL CUT OAT BLUEBERRY PANCAKES	107
SPINACH, MUSHROOM, AND FETA CHEESE SCRAMBLE	108
REFRIGERATOR OVERNIGHT OATMEAL	109
RED VELVET PANCAKES WITH CREAM CHEESE TOPPING	110
PEANUT BUTTER & BANANA BREAKFAST SMOOTHIE	112
MUSHROOM SHALLOT FRITTATA	113
JACK-O-LANTERN PANCAKES	114
MORNING QUINOA	115
FRUIT-N-GRAIN BREAKFAST SALAD	116
FLAX BANANA YOGURT MUFFINS	117
LUNCH RECIPES	118
VEGGIE QUESADILLAS WITH CILANTRO YOGURT DIP	118
SWEET ROASTED BEET & ARUGULA TORTILLA PIZZA	119
PESTO & MOZZARELLA STUFFED PORTOBELLO MUSHROOM CAPS	120
SOUTHWESTERN BLACK BEAN CAKES WITH GUACAMOLE	121
SOUTHWEST STYLE RICE BOWL	122
PEAR, TURKEY AND CHEESE SANDWICH	123
SALMON SALAD PITA	124
FRESH SHRIMP SPRING ROLLS	125
SUNSHINE WRAP	127
HEARTFELT TUNA MELT	128
APPLE-SWISS PANINI	129

California Grilled Veggie Sandwich 130
Chicken, Apple, And Spinach Salad 131
Coconut Shrimp 132
Steamed Spinach 133
Cinnamon Sweet Potatoes 134
Chicken Santa Fe 135
Kung Pao Shrimp 136
Banana Waffles 137
BBQ Baked Beans 138

DINNER RECIPES 140

Beef Stew With Fennel And Shallots 140
Grilled Portobello Mushroom Burger 142
Chicken Brats 144
Asian Pork Tenderloin 146
White Chicken Chili 148
Saucy Chicken 150
Baked Salmon 151
Roasted Turkey 153
Chicken Fried Rice 154
Buffalo & Ranch Chicken Meatloaf 155
Shitake & Snow Peas Quinoa 156
Steamed Mussels 157
Gruyere And Spinach Casserole 159
Honey Garlic Chicken Drumsticks 160
Shrimp Pasta Primavera 161

SALADS & SOUPS RECIPES 163

Easy Shrimp Salad 163
Greek Chicken Salad 165
Chicken Soup 167
Pumpkin Soup 168
Spicy Black Bean Soup 169
Shrimp Soup 171
Kale Salad With Mixed Vegetables 172
Cream Of Corn Soup 173

Clam Soup 174
Curried Quinoa Sweet Potato Salad 175

DESSERTS RECIPES 176

Carrot Cupcakes 176
Stuffed Peaches 177
Dash Diet Doughnuts 179
Berries And Orange Sauce 180
Grapefruit Granita 181
Stewed Plums 182
Whole Wheat Pumpkin Pancakes 183
Pineapple Bowls 185
Tofu Chocolate Cake 186
Chocolate Mousse 187

CONCLUSION 188

Part 1

Introduction

While there are hundreds of different diets out there floating around, you will soon realize that the DASH diet stands on a league of its own!

This particular diet, fully approved and recommended by the U.S Based National Heart, Blood and Lung Institute is a diet that will help you bring out the healthier part of yourself, without having to sacrifice all your favorite foods!

So, what is this diet you ask?

Well, unlike most other diets that focus on losing weight, the DASH diet aims to focus on lowering your blood pressure, which is also represented in the full meaning of the name itself! The word DASH stands for "Dietary Approaches To Stop Hypertension."

And also unlike many other diets, the DASH diet program is the brainchild that was conceived through one of the most intricate and in-depth studies done to date!

The NHLBI worked with five of the most well-respected research centers of that time to come with DASH diet, that was solely designed to tackle the growing hypertension occurrences.

Interesting right?

And the best part is that, if you keep following this diet, not only will you bring down your blood pressure under control, but you will also start losing weight in the long term!

Both of these effects will go to great lengths in keeping your body healthy and trim!

With around 1 billion people all around the world suffering from some form of hypertension, the condition of having high blood pressure levels have never been more severe than it is now!

The core aim of this book is to walk you through the fundamentals of DASH diet while providing you a plethora of amazing recipes that you can make using your Slow Cooker!

So sit back, relax and welcome to the fantastic world of DASH diet Slow Cooking!

Chapter 1: The Fundamentals Of Dash Diet

What Is The Dash Diet?

The DASH (Dietary Approach To Stop Hypertension) diet is a type of healthy dietary eating pattern that was designed to help individuals with hypertension. Despite its primary objective though, following a DASH diet comes with a plethora of other health benefits as well.

Unlike many other diets out there that ask you to get rid of almost all of your favorite food groups! The DASH diet tends to follow a different pathway and asks you to control the "daily serving" of certain foods, as opposed to eliminating them from your regime.

Perhaps one of the more exciting aspects of the Dash Diet is the fact that this particular diet is perhaps one of the very few that have been approved and promoted by the U.S Department of Health and Human Services. So, you can rest easy knowing that this is not just another fad diet!

The DASH Diet tries to tackle the issue of hypertension directly by encouraging you to lower down your sodium intake and eat more foods that are rich in potassium.

Just in case you are wondering, Potassium helps to reduce the effects of excess sodium, which in turn helps to lower down blood pressure, that leads to a significant number of fantastic health benefits.

While the DASH diet primarily focuses on increasing the intake of fruits, vegetables, and low-fat dairy items, you are still allowed to go for meat-based recipes, although in small quantities.

We will look at the dietary requirements of the DASH diet in details later in this chapter, but first, let me walk you through the health benefits of this diet.

Fantastic Dash Diet Health Benefits!

Even though the DASH diet is primarily targeted towards individuals who are struggling with hypertension, there are undoubtedly other health benefits that you should know of. But before talking about the rest, let me discuss the core one first:

Lowers and prevents hypertension

The word "Hypertension" is found in the acronym of DASH itself, which further solidifies the importance of this particular diet when dealing with it.

The DASH diet is the culmination of a large number of different studies that focused on reducing the harmful effects of Hypertension, which makes this particular program extremely efficient at what it does.

To be able to fully appreciate the effectiveness of the diet regarding lowering down Hypertension though, you should have the necessary knowledge of what "Hypertension" actually is.

So in Layman's terms, Hypertension is the shortened term for "High Blood Pressure." When a person experiences this, blood is forcibly pushed through blood vessels at an accelerated rate.

You should know that blood pressure is generally measure using two figures, Systolic and Diastolic Pressure.

When an individual is measured to have a Systolic Pressure of 140mmHg or higher and a Diastolic pressure of 90mmHg or higher, it is diagnosed that they are suffering from Hypertension.

Normal pressure levels are considered to fall at around 120mmHg Systolic and 80mmHg Diastolic.

DASH diet encourages you to eat a good number of fruits and vegetables that are high in Calcium, Magnesium, Potassium and various other antioxidants, that altogether helps to control your Blood Pressure and keep it hovering around the normal levels.

Help lose weight

Despite not being specifically designed for weight loss, Dash Diet does indeed help to trim down your weight through various indirect means.

While DASH diet does not include stress reduction in calorie, it does influence you to fill up your diet with very nutrient dense food as opposed to calorie-rich food; this efficiently helps to shed off few pounds!

Since you will be on a heavy diet of veggies and fruits, you will be consuming lots of fiber, which is also believed to help in weight loss.

Asides from that, the diet also helps to control your appetite since cleaner, and nutrient dense foods will keep you satisfied all throughout the day! Lower food intake will further contribute to weight loss.

Greatly helps to control diabetes

Another significant advantage of the DASH diet is the prevention and control of diabetes. This is an aftereffect of being able to lose your weight in the diet.

And even if you do not have diabetes, the fruits and vegetables chosen for the DASH diet will still help you to keep your calories lower, while making you feel content.

Since Dash Diet helps to eliminate empty carbohydrates and starchy food from your diet, while avoiding simple sugars, a delicate balance between the glucose and insulin level of the body is created that helps to prevent diabetes.

It will help you avoid the temptation of devouring foods that are dredged in sugar or salt and the long run, will help your reverse the insulin resistance!

Asides from the significant three mentioned above, the DASH diet will also:
- Lowers down blood pressure
- Helps to lower down cholesterol levels
- Helps in weight loss (discussed later)
- Gives you a healthier heart
- Helps to prevent Osteoporosis
- Helps to improve Kidney health
- Helps to prevent cancer
- Helps to control Diabetes
- Helps to prevent depression

And those are just the tip of the iceberg!

The Two Types Of Dash

Now that you have a good grasp of what DASH diet is and how it can help you let me briefly talk about just how you can ease into the diet.

So, the first thing that you should know is that there are two different types of DASH diets. Depending on the one that you want to follow, the requirements will slightly vary.

The two types of DASH diets are the standard DASH and the Lower-Sodium DASH diet.

On the standard DASH diet, you are generally allowed to consume 2,300 mg of sodium per day. On the lower-sodium DASH though, you are allowed to go for up to 1,500 mg of sodium.

Both versions of the diets can and will help you to lower down your blood pressure. However, it has been seen that sure people tend to benefit more from the Lower-Sodium version of the diet.

In general, you should aim to follow the Low-Sodium version of the diet if:

- You have chronic kidney diseases
- Suffering from diabetes
- Already have high blood pressure
- Are African American
- Are over 51 years of age

Entering The Dash

Once you have decided which variation of the diet you have chosen for yourself, the next step is to know the general recommendation of the DASH diet, which is as follows:

- 6-8 servings of whole grains (daily)
- 4-5 servings of vegetable (daily)
- 4-5 servings of fruits (daily)
- 2-3 servings of low-fat dairy (Daily)
- 6 or fewer servings of lean meat, poultry or fish (daily)
- 2-3 servings of healthy fats/oils (daily)
- 4-5 servings of nuts, seeds, and legumes (weekly)
- 5 or fewer servings of sweets (weekly)

When considering to design your very own meal plan, you should try to develop a meal plan that would satisfy the above-mentioned requirements as strictly as possible.

And this is where another confusion comes into play. The "Serving" Side.

You should understand that a single serving of rice will not be the same as a single serving of potatoes, even though both of them are from the same group.

Researches have shown that you will be getting a result within just 2 weeks!

Therefore, to make things a little bit easier for you, I have included a few tables that would help you to understand the size of each serving approximately.

How To Kickstart Your Dash Diet

As mentioned earlier, the DASH diet calls for a specific number of servings from various food groups.

Keep in mind that the number of servings will depend on how many calories you need per day, which will change depending on your sex, weight, etc.

An excellent way to calculate your daily calories is to use free online calorie calculators.

Once you have decided on your calorie intake, start off your DASH diet by making incremental and gradual changes.

- An excellent way to start is to limit your sodium to 2,400 mg per day and lower it down eventually
- Once your body has adjusted itself to the change, go for 1,500mg per day (which is about 2/3 spoon)

(Keep in mind that the sodium count includes both the sodium already present in your food as well as any additional salt that you might add)

So to summarize -

- Consume more fruits, low-fat dairy foods, and vegetables
- Try to cut back on foods that are high in cholesterol, saturated fat and trans fat
- Eat whole grain foods, nuts, poultry and fish
- Try to limit down on sodium, sugary drinks, sweets and red meat such as beef/pork, etc.

The Serving Chart

Food Group	Daily Serving (1,200 Calorie Diet)	Daily Serving (2,000 Calorie Diet)	Serving Size	Examples
Whole Grains And Starches	5	7-8	1 ounce dry	- ½ cup cooked whole-

					- wheat pasta - ½ cup cooked brown rice - ½ cup cooked oatmeal
Lean Meat, Poultry, And Fish	4 or fewer	6 or fewer		- 1-ounce fish meat, poultry - 2 egg whites - 1 whole egg	- 1 ounce cooked a turkey breast - 1 scrambled egg
Dairy	2	3		- 8 ounces low-fat milk - 1 cup	- 1 cup skim milk - 1 cup plain

						fat-free yogurt, sour cream cottage cheese	fat-free yogurt
Fruits	3	5				½ cup berries 1 medium fruit ¼ cup dried fruit	½ cup blueberries ½ cup unsweetened pineapple chunks 1 medium apple ¼ cup raisins ¼ cup dried apples 4 ounc

					es lemon
Fats And oil	2	3	<ul><li>1 teaspoon vegetable oil</li><li>1 teaspoon margarine</li><li>1 tablespoon low-fat mayonnaise</li><li>2 tablespoons reduced-fat salad dressing</li></ul>		<ul><li>1 teaspoon extra virgin olive oil</li><li>1 teaspoon soft margarine</li><li>2 tablespoons low-fat vinaigrette</li></ul>
Nuts, Seeds, and Legumes	3 per week	5 per week	<ul><li>2 tablespoons nut butter</li><li>1/3 cup</li></ul>		<ul><li>2 tablespoons unsalted</li></ul>

			• unsalted nuts • 2 tablespoons seeds • ½ cup cooked legumes	• ½ cup unsalted cashew butter • 2 tablespoons chia seeds
Sweets	3 per week	5 per week or fewer	• 1 tablespoon sugar • 2 hard candies • 1 tablespoon jam • 8 ounces sweet beverage	• 1 tablespoon white sugar • 2 peppermint candies • 1 tablespoon

					grape jelly
Sodium Limit	1,500 - 2,300 mg	1,500-2,300 mg		• ½ - 1 teaspoon added salt	

The Food Groups For Dash

To keep things simple, I have divided the food groups into three categories that should guide you during your DASH journey.

Eat as much as you want

- Grains such as Barley, Wheat Bread, Wheat Pasta, etc.
- Meats such as Eggs, Lean Beef, Lean Chicken, Lean Pork
- Seafood such as Fish, Shrimp, and Salmon
- Fruits such as apples, bananas, cherries, grapes, blackberries, mangoes, etc.
- Vegetables such as Artichokes, Broccoli, Brussels, Carrots, Bell Peppers, Green Beans, etc.

Limit Your Servings

- Healthy vegetable oils such as canola, corn, olive, etc.
- Condiments
- Dairy such as Greek yogurt, Skim Milk, Low-Fat Milk, Low-Fat Cheese
- Nuts, Legumes, and Seeds such as Almonds, Cashews, Flax Seeds, Hazel Nuts, Lentils, Pecans, Kidney Beans
- Red Meats

Eat Rarely

- Sweets such as beverages, Jams, Jellies, Sugars, Sweet Yogurt

- Saturated Fats such as Bacon, Cholesterol, Coconuts, Fatty Meats
- Sodium rich foods such as Canned Fruits, Canned Vegetables, Gravy Pizza, etc.

Good Salt Alternatives To Know About

If this is your first time diving into the world of Dash Diet, then you might struggle to find suitable options for salt.

To make life easier for you, below are some of the best salt alternatives that you should consider during your diet.

Sunflower Seeds

Sunflower seeds are fantastic salt alternatives, and they give a sweet nutty and slightly sweet flavor. You may use the seeds raw or roasted.

Fresh Squeezed Lemon

Lemon is believed to a be nice hybrid between citron and bitter orange. These are packed with Vitamin C, which helps to neutralize damaging free radicals from the system.

Onion Powder

For those of you who don't know, Onion powder is a dehydrated and ground spice that is made out of onion bulb. The powder is mostly used for seasoning in many spices! Keep in mind that onion powder and onion salt are two different things.

We are using onion powder here. They sport a nice mix of sweet, spice and bit an earthy flavor.

Black Pepper Powder

The black pepper powder is also a salt alternative that is native to India. You may use them by grinding whole peppercorns!

Cinnamon

Cinnamon is a very popular and savory spice that comes from the inner bark of trees. Two varieties of cinnamon include

Ceylon and Chinese, and they sport a sharp, warm and sweet flavor.

Flavored Vinegar

Fruit infused vinegar or flavored vinegar as we call in our book are mixtures of vinegar that are combined with fruits to give a sweet flavor. These are excellent ingredients to add a bit of flavor to meals without salt. Experimentation might be required to find the perfect fruit blend for you.

As for the process of making the vinegar:

- Wash your fruits and slice them well
- Place ½ a cup of your fruit in a mason jar
- Top them up with white wine vinegar (or balsamic vinegar)
- Allow them to sit for 2 weeks or so
- Strain and use as needed

Awesome Tips For The Journey

And to top it all off! Here are some excellent tips that you should help you along the way.

- Make sure to increase the amount of fresh/frozen fruits and vegetables you consume daily. While you will find a plethora of fruit and veggie based recipes on this book, it is also advised that you develop a habit of munching fruit for either breakfast or snack. Try to make sure that you have a "Balanced" plate, which should include about a half plate of veggies.
- When making your meal plan, make sure to replaced meat-based dishes with various legumes based meals or fish. This would help you to ensure that you can experience the advantages of the diet to its fullest extent.
- Try to go for whole grain products as much as possible. So, Whole Wheat bread, pasta, oats, quinoa, brown rice, etc. are all outstanding options!

- When drinking dairy, try to go for low-fat milk or yogurt. Keep in mind that milk is a very nutritious and healthy alternative to other sugary beverages.
- Make sure to go for a variety of unsalted nuts, seeds a few times per week.
- Try to develop a habit of reading nutritional facts on food labels and compare to find the foods that are made up with the lowest amount of saturated and trans fat.
- Add a serving of veggies at dinner and lunch
- Add a serving of fruit to your meals or such as snacks
- If you wish, then you are allowed to go for low-fat/ skim dairy products as a replacement for full-fat/cream
- If you have a craving for snacks, try to go for unsalted pretzels, raisins or nuts instead of chips or sweets

Chapter 2: Sample 7 Days Meal Plan

Keep in mind that the following meal plan is designed merely to give you an idea as to how you should come up with your plans. Since the caloric requirements vary from one person to the next, the same plan might not apply to you. But the rough structure will be the same.

Be sure to consult with your nutritionist before crafting your plan.

Day	Breakfast	Lunch	Dinner
Sunday	Simple Blueberry Oatmeal	Spicy Baked Cabbage	Sweet Potato Turkey Breast
Monday	Mesmerizing Carrot And Pineapple Mix	Maple Pork Tenderloin	Traditional Black Bean Chili
Tuesday	The "Dashing" Chia Pudding	Herbed Up Salmon	Slow Cooker Mexican Chicken
Wednesday	Simple Blueberry Oatmeal	Auspicious Shrimp Salad	Authentic Greek Pork
Thursday	Mesmerizing Carrot And Pineapple Mix	Spicy Baked Cabbage	Sweet Potato Turkey Breast
Friday	The "Dashing" Chia Pudding	Maple Pork Tenderloin	Traditional Black Bean Chili
Saturday	Simple Blueberry Oatmeal	Herbed Up Salmon	Slow Cooker Mexican Chicken

*If you happen to get the munchies in-between meals, you are allowed to go for some complimentary snacks, as long as they abide by the servings rule and does not exceed your caloric requirements.

Chapter 3: Breakfast Recipes

Simple Blueberry Oatmeal

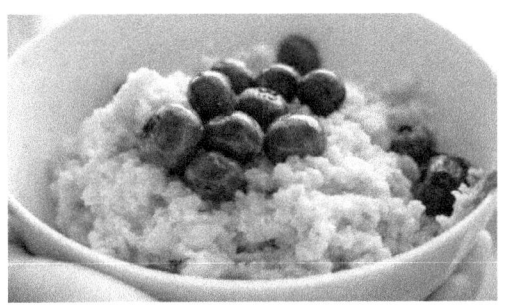

Serving: 4
Prep Time: 10 minutes
Cooking Time: 8 hours
Ingredients:

- 1 cup blueberries
- 1 cup steel cut oats
- 1 cup coconut milk
- 2 tablespoons agave nectar
- ½ teaspoon vanilla extract
- Coconut flakes, garnish

Directions:
1. Grease Slow Cooker with cooking spray
2. Add oats, milk, nectar, blueberries and vanilla
3. Toss well
4. Place lid and cook on LOW for 8 hours
5. Divide between serving bowls and serve

6. Enjoy!

Nutritional Contents:
- Calories: 202
- Fat: 6g
- Carbohydrates: 12g
- Protein: 6g

The "Dashing" Chia Pudding

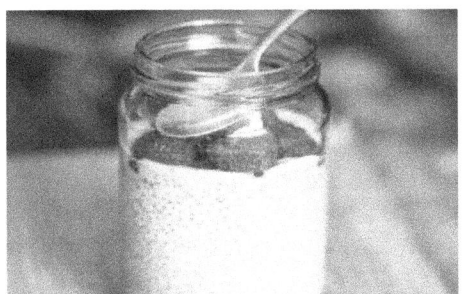

Serving: 4

Prep Time: 10 minutes

Cooking Time: 2 hours

Ingredients:

- ½ cup coconut chia granola
- ½ cup chia seeds
- 2 cups coconut milk
- 2 tablespoons coconut, shredded and sweetened
- ¼ cup maple syrup
- ½ teaspoon cinnamon powder
- 2 teaspoons cocoa powder
- ½ teaspoon vanilla extract

Directions:

1. Add chia granola, chia seeds, coconut milk, maple syrup, coconut, cinnamon, cocoa powder and vanilla to your Slow Cooker
2. Stir and place lid
3. Cook on HIGH for 2 hours
4. Divide between serving bowls and enjoy!

Nutritional Contents:

- Calories: 201
- Fat: 4g
- Carbohydrates: 11g
- Protein: 4g

The Slow Cooker Chicken Omelet

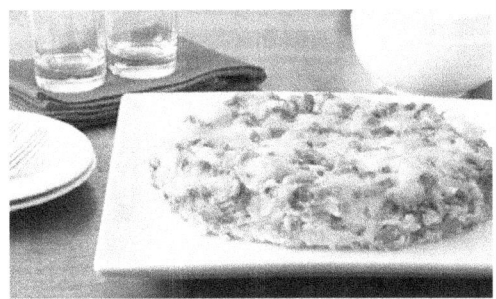

Serving: 2

Prep Time: 10 minutes

Cooking Time: 3 hours

Ingredients:

- 1 ounce rotisserie chicken, shredded
- 1 teaspoon mustard
- 1 tablespoon avocado mayonnaise
- 1 tomato, chopped
- 4 eggs, whisked
- 1 small avocado, pitted, peeled and chopped
- Pepper to taste

Directions:

1. Take a bowl and mix in eggs, chicken, avocado, mayo, mustard and tomato
2. Toss well
3. Transfer mix to Slow Cooker and place lid
4. Cook on LOW for 3 hours
5. Divide between platters and serve
6. Enjoy!

Nutritional Contents:

- Calories: 220
- Fat: 9g
- Carbohydrates: 4g
- Protein: 6g

Tasty Spinach Pie

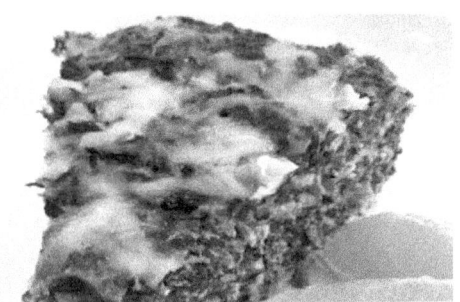

Serving: 2

Prep Time: 10 minutes

Cooking Time: 4 hours

Ingredients:

- 10 ounces spinach
- 2 cups baby Bella mushrooms, chopped
- 1 red bell pepper, chopped
- 1 and ½ cups low-fat cheese, shredded
- 8 whole eggs
- 1 cup coconut cream
- 2 tablespoons chives, chopped
- Pinch of pepper
- ½ cup almond flour
- ¼ teaspoon baking soda

Directions:

1. Take a bowl and add eggs, coconut cream, chives, pepper and whisk well
2. Add almond flour, baking soda, cheese, mushrooms bell pepper, spinach and toss well
3. Grease your cooker and transfer mix to Slow Cooker

4. Place lid and cook on LOW for 4 hours
5. Slice and enjoy!

Nutritional Contents:
- Calories: 201
- Fat: 6g
- Carbohydrates: 8g
- Protein: 5g

Mesmerizing Carrot And Pineapple Mix

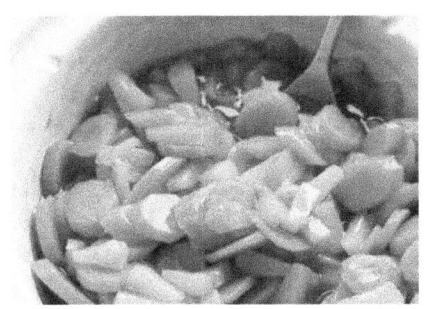

Serving: 10
Prep Time: 10 minutes
Cooking Time: 6 hours
Ingredients:

- 1 cup raisins
- 6 cups water
- 23 ounces natural applesauce
- 2 tablespoons stevia
- 2 tablespoons cinnamon powder
- 14 ounces carrots, shredded
- 8 ounces canned pineapple, crushed
- 1 tablespoon pumpkin pie spice

Directions:

1. Add carrots, applesauce, raisins, stevia, cinnamon, pineapple, pumpkin pie spice to your Slow Cooker and gently stir
2. Place lid and cook on LOW for 6 hours
3. Serve and enjoy!

Nutritional Contents:

- Calories: 179

- Fat: 5g
- Carbohydrates: 15g
- Protein: 4g

Chapter 4: Vegan And Vegetarian Recipes

Traditional Black Bean Chili

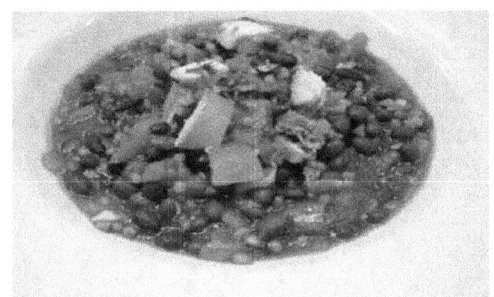

Serving: 4
Prep Time: 10 minutes
Cooking Time: 4 hours
Ingredients:
- 1 and ½ cups red bell pepper, chopped
- 1 cup yellow onion, chopped
- 1 and ½ cups mushrooms, sliced
- 1 tablespoon olive oil
- 1 tablespoon chili powder
- 2 garlic cloves, minced
- 1 teaspoon chipotle chili pepper, chopped
- ½ teaspoon cumin, ground
- 16 ounces canned black beans, drained and rinsed
- 2 tablespoons cilantro, chopped

- 1 cup tomatoes, chopped

Directions:
1. Add red bell peppers, onion, dill, mushrooms, chili powder, garlic, chili pepper, cumin, black beans, tomatoes to your Slow Cooker
2. Stir well
3. Place lid and cook on HIGH for 4 hours
4. Sprinkle cilantro on top
5. Serve and enjoy!

Nutritional Contents:
- Calories: 211
- Fat: 3g
- Carbohydrates: 22g
- Protein: 5g

Amazing Broccoli And Cauliflower Soup

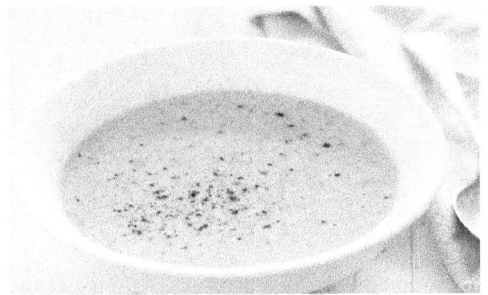

Serving: 4

Prep Time: 10 minutes

Cooking Time: 8 hours

Ingredients:

- 3 cups broccoli florets
- 2 cups cauliflower florets
- 2 garlic cloves, minced
- ½ cup shallots, chopped
- 1 carrot, chopped
- 3 and ½ cups low sodium veggie stick
- Pinch of pepper
- 1 cup fat-free milk
- 6 ounces low-fat cheddar, shredded
- 1 cup non-fat Greek yogurt

Directions:

1. Add broccoli, cauliflower, garlic, shallots, carrot, stock, pepper to your Slow Cooker
2. Stir well and place lid
3. Cook on LOW for 8 hours
4. Add milk and cheese
5. Use an immersion blender to smooth the soup

6. Add yogurt and blend once more
7. Ladle into bowls and enjoy!

Nutritional Contents:

- Calories: 218
- Fat: 11g
- Carbohydrates: 15g
- Protein: 12g

Mesmerizing Lentil Soup

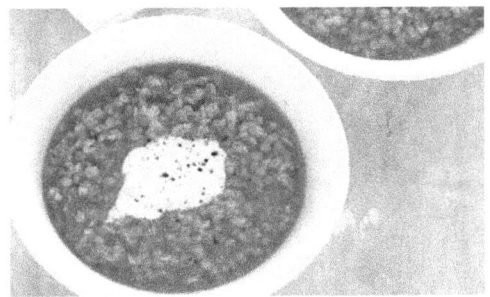

Serving: 4
Prep Time: 10 minutes
Cooking Time: 8 hours
Ingredients:

- 1 pound dried lentils , soaked overnight and rinsed
- 3 carrots, peeled and chopped
- 1 celery stalk, chopped
- 1 onion, chopped
- 6 cups vegetables broth
- 1 and ½ teaspoon garlic powder
- 1 teaspoon ground cumin
- 1 teaspoon smoked paprika
- 1 teaspoon dried thyme
- ¼ teaspoon liquid smoke
- ¼ teaspoon salt
- ¼ teaspoon ground pepper

Directions:

1. Add listed ingredients to Slow Cooker and stir well
2. Place lid and cook for 8 hours on LOW
3. Stir and serve
    4. Enjoy!

Nutritional Contents:
- Calories: 307
- Fat: 1g
- Carbohydrates: 56g
- Protein: 20g

Very Wild Mushroom Pilaf

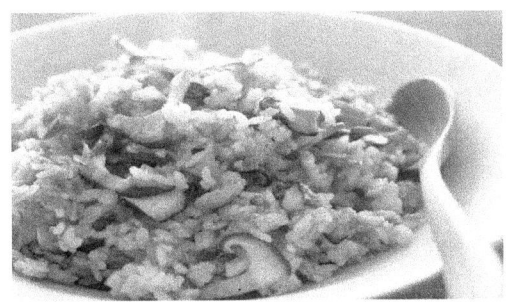

Serving: 4

Prep Time: 10 minutes

Cooking Time: 3 hours

Ingredients:

- 1 cup wild rice
- 2 garlic cloves, minced
- 6 green onions, chopped
- 2 tablespoons olive oil
- ½ pound baby Bella mushrooms
- 2 cups water

Directions:

1. Add rice, garlic, onion, oil, mushrooms and water to your Slow Cooker
2. Stir well until mixed
3. Place lid and cook on LOW for 3 hours
4. Stir pilaf and divide between serving platters
5. Enjoy!

Nutritional Contents:

- Calories: 210
- Fat: 7g
- Carbohydrates: 16g

- Protein: 4g

Spicy Cabbage Dish

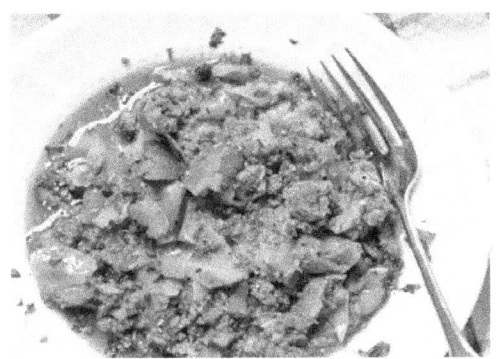

Serving: 4

Prep Time: 10 minutes

Cooking Time: 4 hours

Ingredients:

- 2 yellow onions, chopped
- 10 cups red cabbage, shredded
- 1 cup plums, pitted and chopped
- 1 teaspoon cinnamon powder
- 1 garlic clove, minced
- 1 teaspoon cumin seeds
- ¼ teaspoon cloves, ground
- 2 tablespoons red wine vinegar
- 1 teaspoon coriander seeds
- ½ cup water

Directions:

1. Add cabbage, onion, plums, garlic, cumin, cinnamon, cloves, vinegar, coriander and water to your Slow Cooker
2. Stir well
3. Place lid and cook on LOW for 4 hours

4. Divide between serving platters
5. Enjoy!

Nutritional Contents:
- Calories: 197
- Fat: 1g
- Carbohydrates: 14g
- Protein: 3g

Chapter 5: Side Dish Recipes

Enjoyable Spinach And Bean Medley

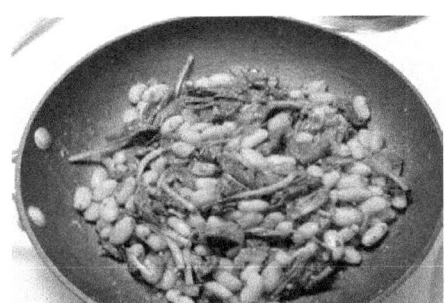

Serving: 4
Prep Time: 10 minutes
Cooking Time: 4 hours
Ingredients:

- 5 carrots, sliced
- 1 and ½ cups great northern beans, dried
- 2 garlic cloves, minced
- 1 yellow onion, chopped
- Pepper to taste
- ½ teaspoon oregano, dried
- 5 ounces baby spinach
- 4 and ½ cups low sodium veggie stock
- 2 teaspoons lemon peel, grated
- 3 tablespoon lemon juice

Directions:

1. Add beans, onion, carrots, garlic, oregano and stock to your Slow Cooker

2. Stir well
3. Place lid and cook on HIGH for 4 hours
4. Add spinach, lemon juice and lemon peel
5. Stir and let it sit for 5 minutes
6. Divide between serving platters and enjoy!

Nutritional Contents:

- Calories: 219
- Fat: 8g
- Carbohydrates: 14g
- Protein: 8g

Edible Okra Mints

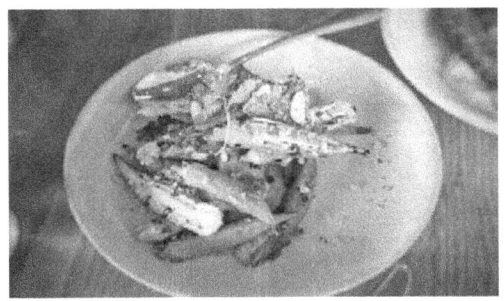

Serving: 3

Prep Time: 10 minutes

Cooking Time: 3 hours

Ingredients:

- 1 pound okra, sliced
- Pepper to taste
- 2 tablespoons mint, chopped
- 2 teaspoons olive oil
- 2 tablespoons low-sodium chicken stock
- 4 green onions, chopped

Directions:

1. Grease Slow Cooker with oil
2. Add okra, pepper, mint, stock and green Onions
3. Stir well
4. Place lid and cook on LOW for 3 hours
5. Divide between plates and serve
6. Enjoy!

Nutritional Contents:

- Calories: 130
- Fat: 1g

- Carbohydrates: 7g
- Protein: 6g

Tantalizing Cauliflower And Dill Mash

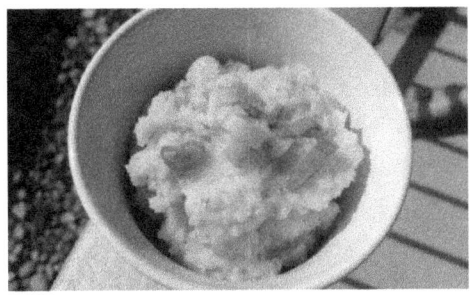

Serving: 6

Prep Time: 10 minutes

Cooking Time: 6 hours

Ingredients:

- 1 cauliflower head, florets separated
- 1/3 cup dill, chopped
- 6 garlic cloves
- 2 tablespoons olive oil
- Pinch of black pepper

Directions:

1. Add cauliflower to Slow Cooker
2. Add dill, garlic and water to cover them
3. Place lid and cook on HIGH for 5 hours
4. Drain the flowers
5. Season with pepper and add oil, mash using potato masher
6. Whisk and serve
7. Enjoy!

Nutritional Contents:

- Calories: 207
- Fat: 4g

- Carbohydrates: 14g
- Protein: 3g

Secret Asian Green Beans

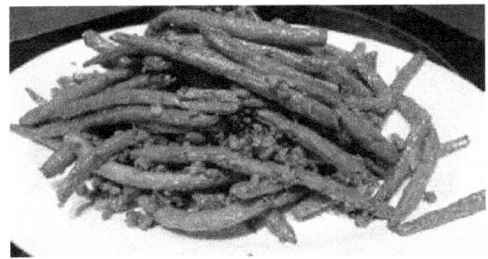

Serving: 10
Prep Time: 10 minutes
Cooking Time: 2 hours
Ingredients:

- 16 cups green beans, halved
- 3 tablespoons olive oil
- ¼ cup tomato sauce, salt-free
- ½ cup coconut sugar
- ¾ teaspoon low sodium soy sauce
- Pinch of pepper

Directions:

1. Add green beans, coconut sugar, pepper tomato sauce, soy sauce, oil to your Slow Cooker
2. Stir well
3. Place lid and cook on LOW for 3 hours
4. Divide between serving platters and serve
5. Enjoy!

Nutritional Contents:

- Calories: 200
- Fat: 4g
- Carbohydrates: 12g
- Protein: 3g

Excellent Acorn Mix

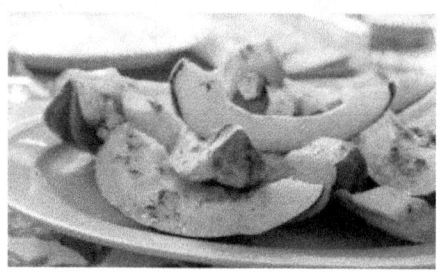

Serving: 10

Prep Time: 10 minutes

Cooking Time: 7 hours

Ingredients:

- 2 acorn squash, peeled and cut into wedges
- 16 ounces cranberry sauce, unsweetened
- ¼ teaspoon cinnamon powder
- Pepper to taste

Directions:

1. Add acorn wedges to your Slow Cooker
2. Add cranberry sauce, cinnamon, raisins and pepper
3. Stir
4. Place lid and cook on LOW for 7 hours
5. Serve and enjoy!

Nutritional Contents:

- Calories: 200
- Fat: 3g
- Carbohydrates: 15g
- Protein: 2g

Chapter 6: Snacks Recipes

Elegant Corn Salad

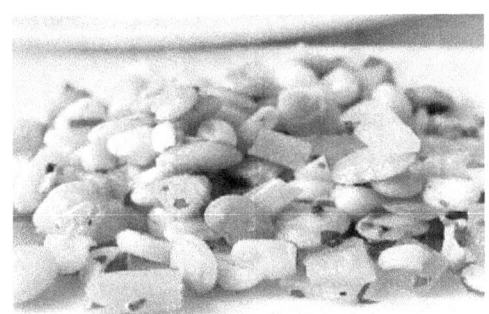

Serving: 6
Prep Time: 10 minutes
Cooking Time: 2 hours
Ingredients:
- 2 ounces prosciutto, cut into strips
- 1 teaspoon olive oil
- 2 cups corn
- 1/2 cup salt –free tomato sauce
- 1 teaspoon garlic, minced
- 1 green bell pepper, chopped

Directions:
1. Grease your Slow Cooker with oil
2. Add corn, prosciutto, garlic, tomato sauce, bell pepper to your Slow Cooker

3. Stir and place lid
4. Cook on HIGH for 2 hours
5. Divide between serving platters and enjoy!

Nutritional Contents:

- Calories: 109
- Fat: 2g
- Carbohydrates: 10g
- Protein: 5g

Quick Asparagus Bite

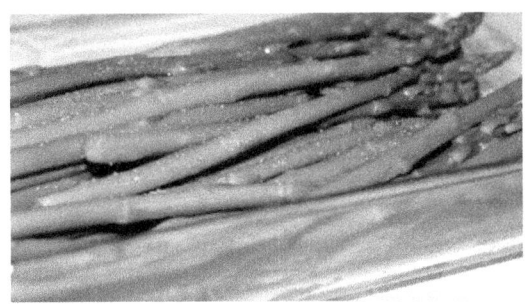

Serving: 4

Prep Time: 10 minutes

Cooking Time: 2 hours

Ingredients:

- 3 cups asparagus spears, halved
- ¼ cup apple cider vinegar
- 1 tablespoon dill
- ¼ cup white wine vinegar
- 2 cloves
- 1 cup water
- 3 garlic cloves, sliced
- ¼ teaspoon red pepper flakes
- 8 black peppercorns
- 1 teaspoon coriander seeds

Directions:

1. Add asparagus, cider vinegar, white vinegar, dill, water, cloves, garlic, pepper flakes, peppercorns and coriander to your Slow Cooker
2. Stir well
3. Place lid and cook on HIGH for 2 hours
4. Drain asparagus and transfer to serving bowl

5. Enjoy!

Nutritional Contents:
- Calories: 90
- Fat: 1g
- Carbohydrates: 7g
- Protein: 2g

Auspicious Italian Shrimp Salad

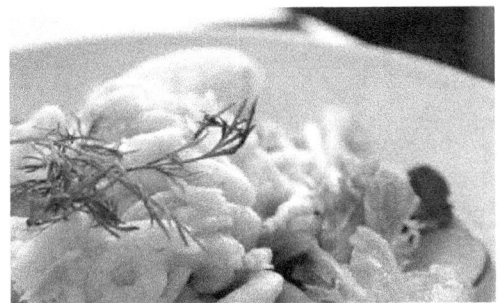

Serving: 8

Prep Time: 10 minutes

Cooking Time: 8 hours

Ingredients:

- 4 cups low-sodium vegetable stock
- 2 tablespoons Italian seasoning
- 1 pound sausage, salt-free and sliced
- Pinch of black pepper
- 2 pounds shrimp ,deveined
- 2 tablespoons parsley, chopped
- 4 tablespoons olive oil

Directions:

1. Add stock, Italian seasoning, sausage, pepper, oil, shrimp to your Slow Cooker
2. Give it a nice toss
3. Place lid and cook on LOW for 8 hours
4. Add parsley, toss again
5. Divide between small serving bowls and enjoy!

Nutritional Contents:

- Calories: 202
- Fat: 3g

- Carbohydrates: 14g
- Protein: 6g

Rickety Nut Mix

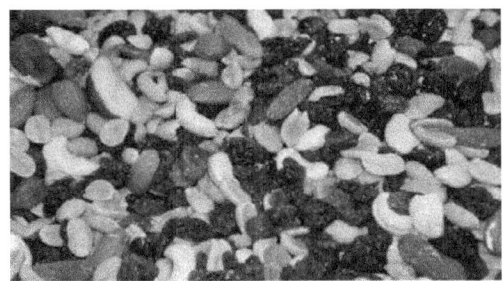

Serving: 20

Prep Time: 10 minutes

Cooking Time: 4 hours

Ingredients:

- 4 tablespoons olive oil
- 1 ounce Italian seasoning
- 1 teaspoon cinnamon powder
- Cayenne pepper to taste
- 2 cups cashews
- 2 cups almonds
- 2 cups walnuts

Directions:

1. Add oil, Italian seasoning, cinnamon to your Slow Cooker
2. Add the nuts and toss them well to coat
3. Place lid and cook on LOW for 4 hours
4. Divide between bowls and serve as snack
5. Enjoy!

Nutritional Contents:

- Calories: 190
- Fat: 4g
- Carbohydrates: 7g

- Protein: 4g

Simple Fish Sticks

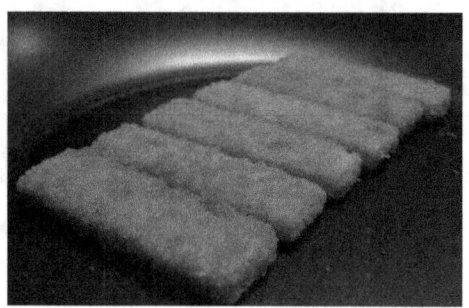

Serving: 4

Prep Time: 10 minutes

Cooking Time: 2 hours

Ingredients:

- 2 whole eggs
- 1 pound white fish fillets, skinless and boneless, cut into medium strips
- Pepper to taste
- 1 cup almond flour
- ¼ teaspoon paprika
- Cooking spray as needed

Directions:

1. Take a bowl and mix flour, pepper, paprika and stir well
2. Take another bowl and crack in the egg, whisk well
3. Dip fish sticks in eggs, then in flour mix
4. Grease your slow cooker with oil
5. Transfer dredged fish sticks to Slow Cooker and spray with cooking spray
6. Place lid and cook on HIGH for 2 hours

7. Serve and enjoy!

Nutritional Contents:
- Calories: 221
- Fat: 2g
- Carbohydrates: 15g
- Protein: 10g

Chapter 7: Poultry Recipes

Hearty Chicken And Veggies

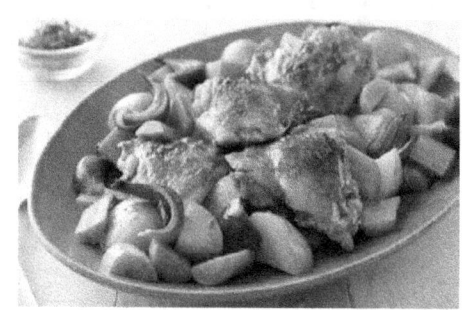

Serving: 4

Prep Time: 10 minutes

Cooking Time: 4 hours

Ingredients:

- 2 pounds chicken breast, skinless and boneless
- 4 cups red potatoes, cubed
- ½ pound green beans, trimmed
- ¼ cup olive oil
- 1/3 cup lemon juice
- 1 teaspoon oregano, dried
- 1 teaspoon cilantro, dried
- Pinch of pepper
- 2 garlic cloves, minced
- ¼ teaspoon onion powder

Directions:

1. Add chicken breast to your Slow Cooker
2. Add green beans and potatoes on top

3. Take a bowl and mix in lemon juice, cilantro, oil, pepper, oregano, garlic and onion powder
4. Mix well
5. Pour the mixture into Slow Cooker
6. Place lid and cook on HIGH for 4 hours
7. Divide chicken and veggies between platters and serve
8. Enjoy!

Nutritional Contents:

- Calories: 211
- Fat: 3g
- Carbohydrates: 16g
- Protein: 5g

All-Time Favorite Pulled Chicken

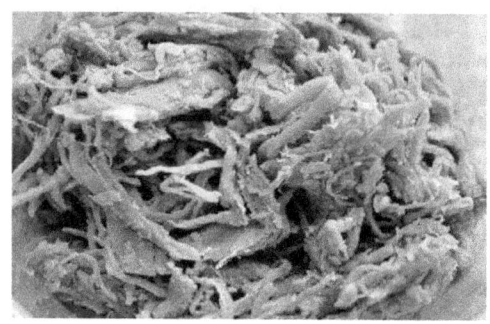

Serving: 4

Prep Time: 10 minutes

Cooking Time: 5 hours

Ingredients:

- 8 ounces tomato sauce, no salt
- 4 ounces green chilies, drained and chopped
- 2 tablespoons honey
- 3 tablespoons cider vinegar
- 1 tablespoon sweet paprika
- 1 tablespoon tomato paste
- 1 tablespoon Worcestershire sauce
- 2 teaspoons dried mustard
- 1 teaspoon chipotle chili, dried and ground
- 2 and ½ pounds chicken thigh, boneless and skinless
- 1 yellow onion, chopped
- 1 garlic clove, minced

Directions:

1. Take a bowl and mix in tomato sauce, honey, green chilies, vinegar, paprika, tomato paste, Worcestershire sauce, chipotle chili, dried mustard and whisk well
2. Pour mix into Slow Cooker

3. Add chicken thighs, onion, garlic and toss
4. Place lid and cook on LOW for 5 hours
5. Shred meat using fork and serve
    6. Enjoy!

Nutritional Contents:

- Calories: 211
- Fat: 3g
- Carbohydrates: 14g
- Protein: 8g

Cool Mediterranean Chicken

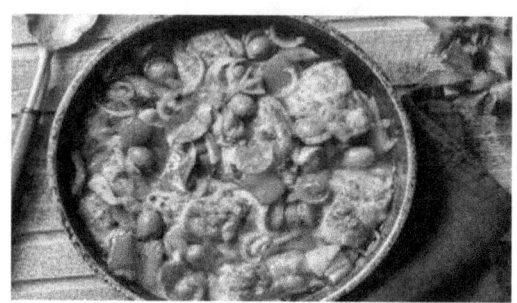

Serving: 4

Prep Time: 10 minutes

Cooking Time: 2 hours 30 minutes

Ingredients:

- 1 pound chicken breast, skinless and boneless
- 2 tomatoes, chopped
- 1 cup low sodium chicken stock
- ½ red bell pepper, chopped
- 1 yellow onion, sliced
- Zest of 1 lemon, grated
- Juice of 1 lemon
- Pepper
- ¾ cup whole wheat orzo
- ½ cup black olives, pitted
- 2 tablespoons scallions, chopped

Directions:

1. Add chicken, tomatoes, bell pepper, onion, zest, lemon juice, pepper to your Slow Cooker
2. Stir
3. Place lid and cook on HIGH for 2 hours
4. Add black olives, orzo and toss

5. Cover and cook on HIGH for 30 minutes more
6. Divide between serving platters and enjoy with a topping of chopped scallions!

Nutritional Contents:

- Calories: 211
- Fat: 5g
- Carbohydrates: 12g
- Protein: 6g

Slow Cooker Mexican Chicken

Serving: 4

Prep Time: 10 minutes

Cooking Time: 7 hours

Ingredients:

- 4 chicken breast, skinless and boneless
- ½ cup water
- 16 ounces chunky salsa
- 1 and ½ tablespoons parsley, chopped
- 1 teaspoon garlic powder
- ½ tablespoon cilantro, chopped
- 1 teaspoon onion powder
- ½ tablespoons oregano, dried
- ½ teaspoon sweet paprika
- 1 teaspoon chili powder
- ½ teaspoon cumin, ground
- Black pepper to taste

Directions:

1. Add water to your Slow Cooker
2. Add chicken breast, parsley, salsa, garlic powder, onion powder, cilantro, oregano, chili powder, paprika, cumin and pepper
3. Gently stir
4. Place lid and cook LOW for 7 hours
5. Divide the whole mix between serving platters and enjoy!

Nutritional Contents:

- Calories: 200
- Fat: 4g
- Carbohydrates: 12g
- Protein: 9g

Sweet Potato Turkey Breast

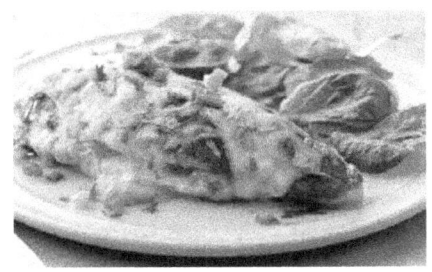

Serving: 4

Prep Time: 10 minutes

Cooking Time: 8 hours

Ingredients:

- 3 pounds turkey breast, bone in
- 3 sweet potatoes, cut into wedges
- 1 cup dried cherries, pitted
- 2 white onion, cut into wedges
- 1/3 cup water
- 1 teaspoon onion powder
- 1 teaspoon garlic powder
- 1 teaspoon parsley flakes
- 1 teaspoon sage, dried
- 1 teaspoon thyme, dried
- 1 teaspoon paprika, dried
- Pepper to taste

Directions:

1. Add turkey breast to Slow Cooker

2. Add sweet potatoes, cherries water, onion, parsley, garlic, onion powder, thyme, sage, paprika and pepper to your Slow Cooker as well
3. Gently stir
4. Place lid and cook on LOW for 8 hours
5. Discard bones from turkey breast, carefully slice the meat
6. Divide between plates and serve with vegetables and cherries
7. Enjoy!

Nutritional Contents:

- Calories: 220
- Fat: 5g
- Carbohydrates: 8g
- Protein: 15g

Chapter 8: Meat Recipes

Healthy And Juicy Pork Roast

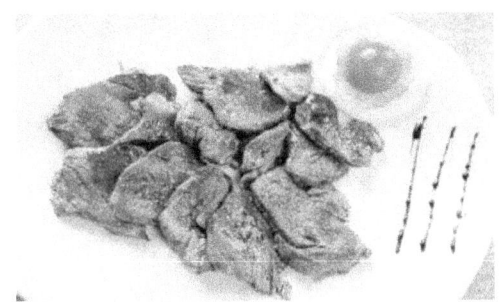

Serving: 8
Prep Time: 10 minutes
Cooking Time: 8 hours
Ingredients:

- 2 pounds pork shoulder roast, boneless
- 1/3 cup low sodium vegetable stock
- ½ teaspoon garlic powder
- 1 tablespoon sage, dried
- ¼ cup balsamic vinegar
- 1 tablespoon low sodium Worcestershire sauce
- 1 tablespoon honey

Directions:

1. Add roast to Slow Cooker
2. Pour stock
3. Take a bowl and mix garlic powder, vinegar, Worcestershire sauce, honey and whisk well

4. Pour mix into Slow Cooker
5. Place lid and cook on LOW for 8 hours
6. Shred meat and serve with the cooking juice
7. Enjoy!

Nutritional Contents:

- Calories: 214
- Fat: 12g
- Carbohydrates: 5g
- Protein: 21g

Authentic Greek Pork

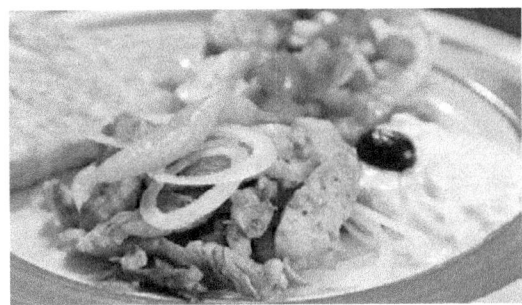

Serving: 6

Prep Time: 15 minutes + 1 day

Cooking Time: 8 hours

Ingredients:

- 3 pounds pork shoulder, boneless
- ¼ cup olive oil
- 2 teaspoons oregano, dried
- ¼ cup lemon juice
- 2 teaspoons mustard
- 2 teaspoons mint
- 6 garlic clove, minced
- Pepper to taste

Directions:

1. Take a bowl and add lemon juice, oil, oregano, mint, garlic, mustard, pepper and mix well
2. Rub the mixture all over pork and cover, refrigerate for 1 day
3. Transfer to Slow Cooker alongside marinade and place lid
4. Cook on LOW for 8 hours
5. Slice and serve
    6. Enjoy!

Nutritional Contents:
- Calories: 260
- Fat: 4g
- Carbohydrates: 14g
- Protein: 8g

Foreign Moroccan Lamb Dish

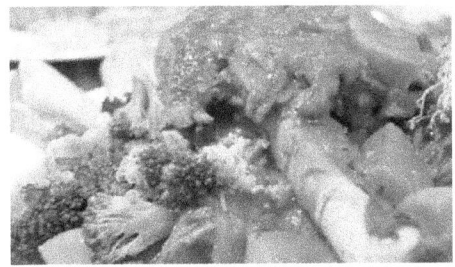

Serving: 6

Prep Time: 15 minutes

Cooking Time: 8 hours

Ingredients:

- 1 pound lamb shoulder, trimmed and cut into 1 inch cubes
- 2 cups beef broth
- 2 cups cherry tomatoes
- 2 onions, sliced
- 1 tablespoon fresh ginger, grated
- 2 teaspoons ground cumin
- 1 teaspoon garlic powder
- ½ teaspoon ground cinnamon
- 1/4 teaspoon black pepper
- 3 cups cooked whole-wheat couscous
- ¼ cup fresh cilantro, chopped

Directions:

1. Add lamb, broth, tomatoes, onions, ginger, cumin, garlic powder, pepper and cinnamon to your Slow Coker
2. Stir well
3. Place lid and cook on LOW for 8 hours
4. Skim any excess fat from the surface
5. Serve over couscous with a garnish cilantro

6. Enjoy!

Nutritional Contents:
- Calories: 353
- Fat: 6g
- Carbohydrates: 45g
- Protein: 28g

Maple Pork Tenderloin

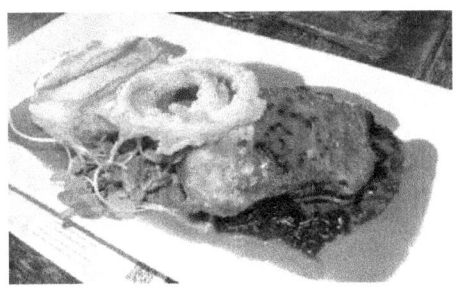

Serving: 4

Prep Time: 10 minutes

Cooking Time: 8 hours

Ingredients:

- Pinch of nutmeg, ground
- 2 pounds pork tenderloin, trimmed
- 4 apples, cored and sliced
- 2 tablespoons maple syrup

Directions:

1. Add half of apples to Slow Cooker
2. Sprinkle nutmeg, add pork tenderloin
3. Top with remaining apples
4. Drizzle maple syrup
5. Place lid and cook on LOW for 8 hours
6. Slice pork tenderloin, divide between plates and serve with apple slices
7. Drizzle the cooking liquid on top
8. Enjoy!

Nutritional Contents:

- Calories: 240
- Fat: 4g

- Carbohydrates: 14g
- Protein: 14g

Juicy Hungarian Goulash

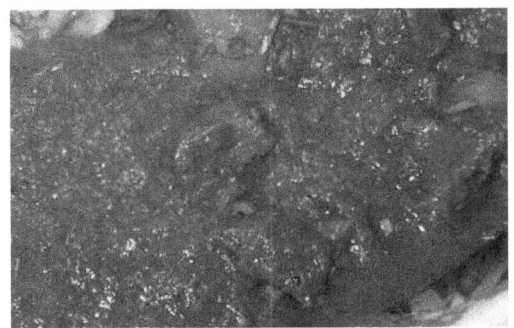

Serving: 6

Prep Time: 15 minutes

Cooking Time: 8 hours

Ingredients:

- 2 cups beef broth
- 1 tablespoon cornstarch
- 1 pound stew beef, trimmed and cut into 1 inch cubes
- 2 onions, sliced
- 3 carrots, peeled and sliced
- ¼ cup tomato paste
- 2 tablespoons smoked paprika
- 1 teaspoon garlic powder
- 3 cups cooked quinoa

Directions:

1. Take a small bowl and add broth and cornstarch
2. Mix well
3. Add mix to slow cooker
4. Add beef, onions, carrots, tomato paste, paprika, garlic powder
5. Stir well
6. Place lid and cook on LOW for 8 hours

7. Skim any excess fat and discard
8. Serve over cooked quinoa and enjoy!

Nutritional Contents:

- Calories: 321
- Fat: 8g
- Carbohydrates: 39g
- Protein: 25g

Chapter 9: Dessert Recipes

Hearty Pineapple Pudding

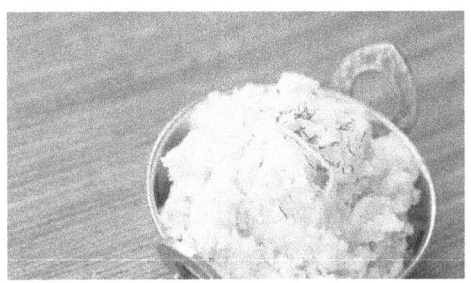

Serving: 4
Prep Time: 10 minutes
Cooking Time: 5 hours
Ingredients:
- 1 teaspoon baking powder
- 1 cup coconut flour
- 3 tablespoons stevia
- 3 tablespoons avocado oil
- ½ cup coconut milk
- ½ cup pecans, chopped
- ½ cup pineapple, chopped
- ½ cup lemon zest, grated
- 1 cup pineapple juice, natural

Directions:
1. Grease Slow Cooker with oil
2. Take a bowl and mix in flour, stevia, baking powder, oil, milk, pecans, pineapple, lemon zest, pineapple juice and stir well

3. Pour the mix into Slow Cooker
4. Place lid and cook on LOW for 5 hours
5. Divide between bowls and serve
6. Enjoy!

Nutritional Contents:

- Calories: 188
- Fat: 3g
- Carbohydrates: 14g
- Protein: 5g

Crunchy Almond Chocolate Bars

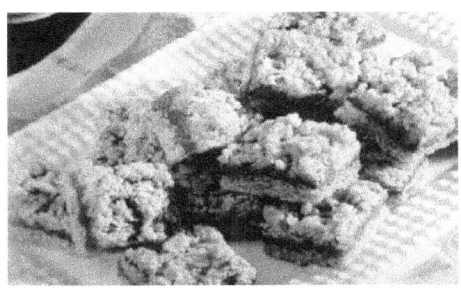

Serving: 12

Prep Time: 10 minutes

Cooking Time: 2 hours 30 minutes

Ingredients:

- 1 egg white
- ¼ cup coconut oil, melted
- 1 cup coconut sugar
- ½ teaspoon vanilla extract
- 1 teaspoon baking powder
- 1 and ½ cps almond meal
- ½ cup dark chocolate chips

Directions:

1. Take a bowl and add sugar, oil, vanilla extract, egg white, almond flour, baking powder and mix it well
2. Fold in chocolate chips and stir
3. Line slow cooker with parchment paper
4. Grease
5. Add cookie mix and press on bottom
6. Place lid and cook on LOW for 2 hours 30 minutes
7. Take cookie sheet out and let it cool
8. Cut in bars and enjoy!

Nutritional Contents:
- Calories: 200
- Fat: 2g
- Carbohydrates: 13g
- Protein: 6g

Healthy Berry Cobbler

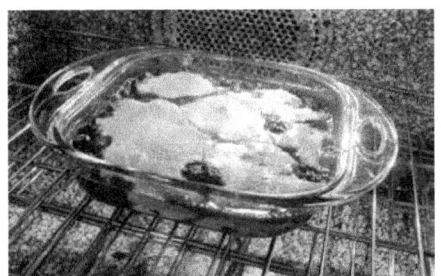

Serving: 8

Prep Time: 10 minutes

Cooking Time: 2 hours 30 minutes

Ingredients:

- 1 and ¼ cups almond flour
- 1 cup coconut sugar
- 1 teaspoon baking powder
- ½ teaspoon cinnamon powder
- 1 whole egg
- ¼ cup low-fat milk
- 2 tablespoons olive oil
- 2 cups raspberries
- 2 cups blueberries

Directions:

1. Take a bowl and add almond flour, coconut sugar, baking powder and cinnamon
2. Stir well
3. Take another bowl and add egg, milk, oil, raspberries, blueberries and stir
4. Combine both of the mixtures
5. Grease your Slow Cooker

6. Pour the combined mixture into your Slow Cooker and cook on HIGH for 2 hours 30 minutes
7. Divide between serving bowls and enjoy!

Nutritional Contents:
- Calories: 250
- Fat: 4g
- Carbohydrates: 30g
- Protein: 3g

Tasty Poached Apples

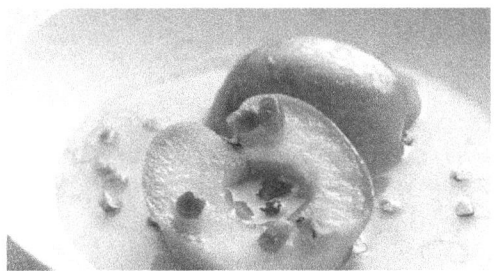

Serving: 8

Prep Time: 10 minutes

Cooking Time: 2 hours 30 minutes

Ingredients:

- 6 apples, cored, peeled and sliced
- 1 cup apple juice, natural
- 1 cup coconut sugar
- 1 tablespoon cinnamon powder

Directions:

1. Grease Slow Cooker with cooking spray
2. Add apples, sugar, juice, cinnamon to your Slow Cooker
3. Stir gently
4. Place lid and cook on HIGH for 4 hours
5. Serve cold and enjoy!

Nutritional Contents:

- Calories: 180
- Fat: 5g
- Carbohydrates: 8g
- Protein: 4g

Heart Warming Cinnamon Rice Pudding

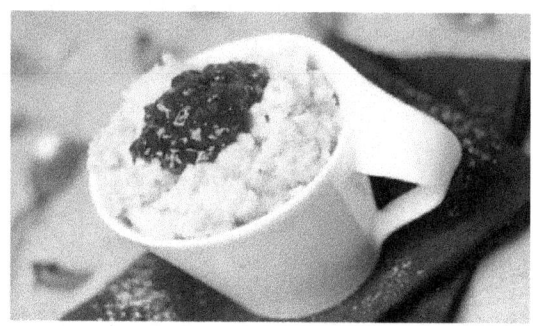

Serving: 4

Prep Time: 10 minutes

Cooking Time: 5 hours

Ingredients:

- 6 and ½ cups water
- 1 cup coconut sugar
- 2 cups white rice
- 2 cinnamon sticks
- ½ cup coconut, shredded

Directions:

1. Add water, rice, sugar, cinnamon and coconut to your Slow Cooker
2. Gently stir
3. Place lid and cook on HIGH for 5 hours
4. Discard cinnamon
5. Divide pudding between dessert dishes and enjoy!

Nutritional Contents:

- Calories: 173

- Fat: 4g
- Carbohydrates: 9g
- Protein: 4g

Chapter 10: Fish Recipes

Herbed Up Salmon

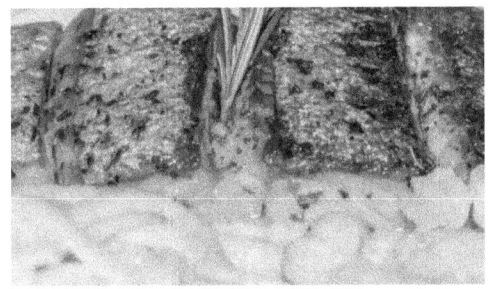

Serving: 4

Prep Time: 10 minutes

Cooking Time: 2 hours 30 minutes

Ingredients:

- 2 garlic cloves, minced
- 4 salmon fillets, boneless and skin on
- 1 cup cilantro, chopped
- 3 tablespoons lime juice
- 1 tablespoon olive oil
- Black pepper to taste

Directions:

1. Grease Slow Cooker with oil
2. Add salmon fillets, garlic, cilantro, lime juice, pepper to your Slow Cooker
3. Place lid and cook on LOW for 2 hours 30 minutes
4. Divide between serving platters

5. Drizzle cilantro sauce
6. Enjoy!

Nutritional Contents:

- Calories: 220
- Fat: 3g
- Carbohydrates: 14g
- Protein: 8g

The Asian Salmon Delight

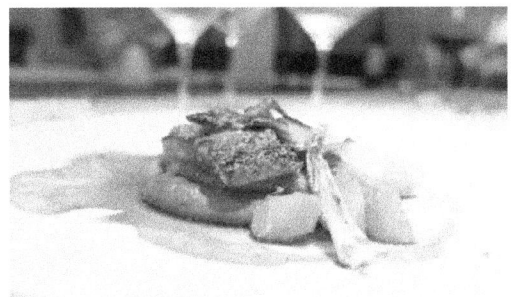

Serving: 2

Prep Time: 10 minutes

Cooking Time: 3 hours

Ingredients:

- 2 medium salmon fillets, boneless
- Pepper to taste
- 2 tablespoons low sodium soy sauce
- 2 tablespoons maple syrup
- 16 ounces mixed broccoli and cauliflower florets
- 2 tablespoons lemon juice
- 1 teaspoon sesame seeds

Directions:

1. Add cauliflower, broccoli florets to Slow Cooker
2. Top with Salmon
3. Take a bowl and mix in maple syrup, soy sauce, lemon juice and whisk well
4. Pour over salmon mix
5. Season with pepper, sprinkle sesame seeds on top
6. Place lid and cook on LOW for 3 hours
7. Divide between plates and serve
    8. Enjoy!

Nutritional Contents:

- Calories: 230
- Fat: 4g
- Carbohydrates: 13g
- Protein: 8g

The Lemon And Spinach "Trout" Dish

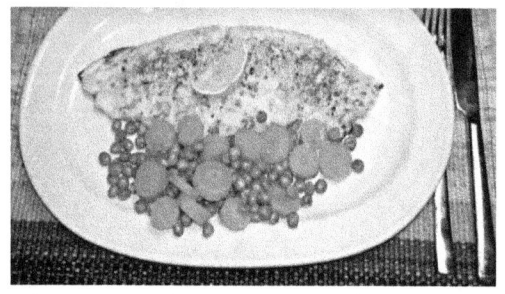

Serving: 4

Prep Time: 10 minutes

Cooking Time: 2 hours

Ingredients:

- 2 lemons, sliced
- ¼ cup low sodium chicken stock
- Pepper to taste
- 2 tablespoons dill, chopped
- 12 ounces spinach
- 4 medium trout

Directions:

1. Add stock to your Slow Cooker
2. Gently place fish
3. Season with pepper
4. Top with lemon slices, spinach and dill

5. Place lid and cook on HIGH for 2 hours
6. Prepare servings by dividing fish, spinach and lemon between serving platters
7. Enjoy!

Nutritional Contents:

- Calories: 240
- Fat: 5g
- Carbohydrates: 9g
- Protein: 14g

Simple Slow Cooker Tuna

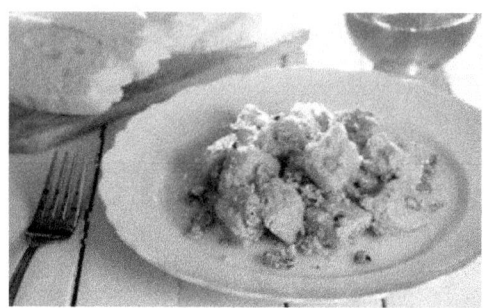

Serving: 2

Prep Time: 10 minutes

Cooking Time: 4 hours 10 minutes

Ingredients:

- ½ pound tuna loin, cubed
- 1 garlic clove, minced
- 4 jalapeno peppers, chopped
- 1 cup olive oil
- 3 red chili peppers, chopped
- 2 teaspoons black peppercorn, ground
- Pepper to taste

Directions:

1. Add oil to your Slow Cooker
2. Grease it well
3. Add chili pepper, jalapenos, peppercorns, pepper, garlic to Slow Cooker and whisk it well
4. Place lid and cook on LOW for 4 hours
5. Add tuna and toss
6. Place lid and cook on HIGH for 10 minutes more
7. Divide between serving platters and enjoy!

Nutritional Contents:

- Calories: 190
- Fat: 4g
- Carbohydrates: 10g
- Protein: 4g

Conclusion

I can't express how honored I am to think that you found my book interesting and informative enough to read it all through to the end.

I thank you again for purchasing this book and I hope that you had as much fun reading it as I had writing it.

I bid you farewell and encourage you to move forward with your Dash Diet Slow Cooking Journey!

Patr 2

Introduction

The DASH diet is as a result of medical professionals who worked for years on dietary strategies for sustaining normal blood pressure levels and weight loss. The DASH Diet was therefore tested, trusted and approved to reduce blood pressure in both individuals who are healthy and those suffering from hypertension by nutritionists and medical professionals. Since our health is greatly affected by what we eat, the right change in diet can change your life for greatness, and DASH Diet is the way to go. We help maintain our blood pressure when we eat plenty of vegetables, fruits and lean proteins like chicken and fish while minimizing the intake of red meat, processed sugars, salt and unhelpful fats.

The DASH Diet does not only help in lowering blood pressure, but it also aids in weight loss, prevention of related heart diseases, cancer and diabetes due to high intake of vegetables and fruits. The art of minimizing blood pressure naturally without being hospitalized or under medication is attractive to everyone while we enjoy the dash diet whole meals. It is more fulfilling.

Such a cheap combination of dieting practices end up among the most praise dieting approaches all over, and so if you would wish to lose weight while lowering your blood pressure, I will recommend for you the DASH Diet. Do so by counting the calories, and you will love it.

This DASH Diet cookbook is designed to help you in planning for your healthy future. The recipes are clear and easy to follow with simple ingredients that won't give you a hard time. Once you understand and follow them promptly, you will be amazed by the outcome. Have a great time with DASH Diet!

What Is Dash Diet?

DASH diet stands for Dietary Approaches to Stop Hypertension. It is a simple diet that is highly appreciated as it promotes healthy living. The diet was designed majorly to lower blood pressure and reduce risks involved in heart-related illness, cancer, diabetes, osteoporosis, stroke, and healthy weight loss.

The diet enables you to reduce sodium intake and start eating healthier foods that have useful nutrients. The DASH Diet has two options though you need to consult with the doctor before you start off.

During the first phase, you can consume up to 2300 mg of sodium per day while the second phase, the sodium rate lowers to 1500 mg per day.

Both versions of the diet include plenty of vegetables, low-fat and non-fat dairy, fruits, whole grains and lean protein like poultry, fish or seafood in your diet. The major thing to keep in mind is that you not only need to reduce the amount of sodium intake but also sugar and fat. All you need to do is to find products and ingredients that have useful nutrients like magnesium, potassium, or calcium.

If you are on a DASH Diet, you can take whole grains like oats, cereals, quinoa, rice, pasta or bread. The basic thing you need to remember is that you must not combine them with other products having lots of fat or cholesterol. The vegetables should be in plenty. Mostly potatoes, spinach, tomatoes, turnips, pumpkin, green beans among others. If you choose frozen veggies, ensure they don't have added salt.

One of the great advantages of DASH Diet is that you can consume a wide range of plenty fruits as you wish. They include cherries, bananas, melons, pineapples, apples, and dates among others.

You can take low-fat dairy milk, yogurt, buttermilk, cheese and some butter. Ensure they are the right ones specifically for DASH Diet. When taking meat, it is advisable either you grill, broil or bakes instead of frying.

When it comes to spices and seasoning, salt should be used sparingly or use spices like, bay leaves, basil, cinnamon, cardamom, ginger powder, garlic powder, and pepper.

Avoid using canned products as much as possible since most of them contain a lot of salt. If you must use, ensure you read the label before purchasing.

Basic Rules & Benefits Of Dash Diet

In order for DASH Diet to be fulfilling, some considerations have to be put in place. They include:

Lifestyle change:

The DASH Diet isn't a short period, but it is meant to be practiced entirely in your life. You should get ready for such changes.

Ensure you add a low-fat dairy product at every meal to reach 3 servings of required dairy products.

Fresh vegetables with low sodium should be chosen. Avoid canned or frozen vegetables, or if need be, ensure no salt is added.

Ensure you read food labels thoroughly and choose the ones with low sodium and low fat. If you crave for something sweet, go for dried fruit.

Use some food substitutes for various food items like whole wheat pasta or brown rice instead of normal noodles and white rice. For desserts, go for fruits or other healthy foods instead of sweet and products with high calories.

Remember to exercise always as part of a healthy lifestyle. Taking DASH Diet is just part of living healthy. Being active and planning regular exercise to accompany your diet is very important.

Use a food journal to aid you to keep track of what you are supposed to eat.

Ensure that you choose fulfilling meals.

The feeling of being satisfied after meal intake is known as being satiated, and satiety is known to suppress the feeling of hunger for a long time. When we take meals and drink, our bodies produce different chemicals and signal as the food and drink are being digested, this is why we feel 'full' or satiated after a healthy meal.

In general, foods high in protein make us feel full for long, to curb the situation, try including some protein at least every other meal through the day.

Avoid the use of alcohol as it stimulates and magnifies appetite within a short term.

Minimize liquid calories by cutting sugary drinks to a low. Cut them off if possible.

Try to consume food that is high water like soups. This enables us to maintain our usual portion size while minimizing the overall calories content of the meal.

Prepare meals from scratch as it allows for greater control over what we need to eat.

Reduce Your Sodium Intake:

As much as the human body requires sodium to be alive and active, it is also needed to maintain balanced levels of hydration, muscle contraction-relaxation, and to transmit nerve signals and impulses. However, it doesn't take much sodium to overdo it, and the sodium levels contained within our daily salt intake are where a lot of high blood pressure problems starts. Less sodium in the DASH Diet helps lower hypertension or even completely avoid blood pressure related problems.

In the original DASH Diet research, sodium intake was minimized to 1 teaspoon on a daily basis. Over time this can usually be lowered to around 2/3 tsp.

Here are some simple steps you can take to minimize your sodium and salt intake:

- Ensure you read the label
- Make up your personal meal plan
- Prepare your meals
- Try on different spices
- Do away with junk food
- **Avoid canned food**

Increase Magnesium, Calcium and Potassium Intake:

The above-named minerals play a vital role in the proper functioning of our bodies. Minerals and nutrients are known to be electrolytes as they cooperate to help in regulating many of the body functioning among the functions being bone and muscle development, maintaining nerve and heart signals. On a daily basis, we lose the electrolytes through sweating and going the washroom. It is important therefore to refill regularly and take plenty of water.

The 3 most important minerals are:

Magnesium – helps in the functioning of the nerve, bone and strength development. It as well assists in keeping a healthy and proper rhythm of the heart.

Calcium – aids in muscle contractions, bone development, cell division and blood clotting.

Potassium – helps in maintaining stable blood pressure levels as well as heart contractions and muscle function.

When we lack magnesium, calcium, and potassium, we face electrolyte imbalance which can cause symptoms like muscle cramps, anxiety, general weakness, body fluids imbalance, unstable blood pressure, joint pain, difficulty in concentrating, heart palpitations, insomnia, short illnesses, high temperature changes, tiredness, dizziness, frequent thirst among others.

Another rule for dieting is to increase fiber intake to avoid complications like bloating, low blood sugar levels, diarrhea, and constipation among other problems.

When on DASH Diet, replace sugary cravings with fruits, honey, trail mix, smoothies, chewing gum, jam or jelly.

Reduce caffeine intake and drink lots of liquids.

Take nuts like walnuts, cashew nuts, pecans, almonds, hazelnuts, pistachios as snacks. They are the best for dash dieting.

Benefits of DASH Diet

With the rising number of diets all over, it can be hard to distinguish to identify the one that will suit your body and lifestyle. For DASH Diet, it was meant mostly for hypertension or high blood pressure patients.

It is beneficial when it comes to losing weight and reduction of blood pressure.

It is versatile to those who make it as part of their daily routine. When it comes to sodium intake, there are two options. First, those who want a simple decrease in their sodium intake can opt for 2,300 milligrams as a standard level consumption and for those who want to eliminate more of sodium will take 1500 milligrams per day.

Another advantage of the DASH Diet is that it is not totally restrictive compared to other diets. It can be done in two phases, the first one approximating to two weeks. During this period, the dieter must do away with starchy meals as much as possible. This helps to lose the maximum amount of belly fat. In the second phase, healthy starches are re-introduced to the diet with the idea that the body will have already boosted metabolism to handle them. The dieters are advised to stick to phase two as they continue to lose weight.

Another advantage is that stage two is comfortable with the eating patterns in which people have already been relying on simple switches like empty to whole grains and snacks high I protein. The rate of sacrifice is minimal compared to what you get, the benefits.

Breakfast Recipes

Very Berry Muesli

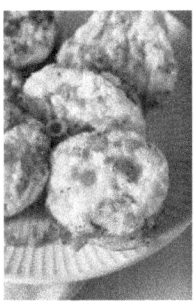

Preparation time: 6 mins

Servings: 2

Nutritional Information: 195 Calories, 6g Protein, 31g Carbs, 4g Fat, 108mg sodium

Ingredients:
- 1 c. oats
- 1 c. fruit flavored yogurt
- ½ c. milk
- 1/8 tsp. salt
- ½ c. dried raisins
- ½ c. chopped apple
- ½ c. frozen blueberries
- **¼ c. chopped walnuts**

Directions:
1. Combine your yogurt, salt, and oats together in a medium bowl, mix well, and then cover the mixture tightly.
2. Allow to rest in the refrigerator for at least 6 hours. Add your raisins, and apples the gently fold.
3. **Top with walnuts and serve. Enjoy!**

Veggie Quiche Muffins

Preparation time: 10 mins

Servings: 12

Nutritional Information: 58.5 Calories, 5.1 g Protein, 2.9 g Carbs, 3.2 g Fat, 304mg sodium

Ingredients:
- ¾ c. shredded cheddar
- 1 c. chopped green onion
- 1 c. chopped broccoli
- 1 c. diced tomatoes
- 2 c. milk
- 4 eggs
- 1 c. pancake mix
- 1 tsp. oregano
- ½ tsp. salt
- **½ tsp. pepper**

Directions:
1. Set your oven to preheat to 375 degrees F, and lightly grease a 12-cup muffin tin with oil. Sprinkle your tomatoes, broccoli, onions, and cheddar into your muffin cups.
2. Combine your remaining ingredients in a medium bowl, whisk to combine then pour evenly on top of your veggies.
3. **Set to bake in your preheated oven for about 40 minutes or until golden brown. Allow to cool slightly (about 5 minutes) then serve. Enjoy!**

Turkey Sausage And Mushroom Strata

Preparation time: 10 mins

Servings: 12

Nutritional Information: 288 Calories, 24.3g Protein, 18.2g Carbs, 12.4g Fat, 730mg sodium.

Ingredients:
- 8 oz. cubed ciabatta bread
- 12 oz. chopped turkey sausage
- 2 c. milk
- 4 oz. shredded cheddar
- 3 large eggs
- 12 oz. egg substitute
- ½ c. chopped green onion
- 1 c. diced mushrooms
- ½ tsp. paprika
- ½ tsp. pepper
- **2 tbsp. grated parmesan cheese**

Directions:
1. Set oven to preheat to 400 degrees F.
2. Lay your bread cubes flat on a baking tray and set it to toast for about 8 min. Meanwhile, add a skillet over medium heat with sausage, and allow to cook, while stirring, until fully brown and crumbled.
3. In a large bowl add salt, pepper, paprika, parmesan cheese, egg substitute, eggs, cheddar cheese, and milk, then whisk to combine.
4. Add in your remaining ingredients and toss well to incorporate.
5. Transfer mixture to a large baking dish (preferably a 9x13-inch) then tightly cover and allow to rest in the refrigerator overnight.

6. Set your oven to preheat to 350 degrees, remove the cover from your casserole and set to bake until fully cooked and golden brown.
7. **Slice and serve.**

Summer Breakfast Quinoa Bowls

Preparation time: 5 mins

Servings: 2

Nutritional Information: 180 Calories, 4.5 g Protein, 36g Carbs, 4g Fat,136mg sodium

Ingredients:
- 1 sliced peach
- 1/3 c. quinoa
- 1 c. low fat milk
- ½ tsp. vanilla extract
- 2 tsp. brown sugar
- 12 raspberries
- 14 blueberries
- **2 tsp. honey**

Directions:
1. Add brown sugar, 2/3 cup milk, and quinoa to a saucepan, and stir to combine.
2. Bring to a boil over medium heat then cover and reduce heat to a low simmer.
3. Continue to cook for about 20 minutes (you should be able to fluff quinoa with a fork).
4. Grease and preheat your grill to medium and grill your peach slices for about a minute per side then set aside.
5. Reheat your remaining milk in the microwave and set aside.
6. **Split your cooked quinoa evenly between 2 serving bowls and top evenly with your remaining ingredients. Enjoy!**

Strawberry Breakfast Sandwich

Preparation time: 5 mins

Servings: 4

Nutritional Information: 180 Calories, 2.0g Protein, 9.0g Carbs, 16g Fat, 277mg sodium.

Ingredients:
- 8 oz. cream cheese
- 1 tbsp. honey
- 1 tbsp. grated lemon zest
- 4 sliced English muffins
- **2 c. sliced strawberries**

Directions:
1. Add your honey, lemon zest, and cheese to a food processor, and process until fully incorporated.
2. Use your cheese mixture to spread on your English muffins as you would butter.
3. **Top with strawberries. Enjoy!**

Steel Cut Oat Blueberry Pancakes

Preparation time: 5 mins

Servings: 4

Nutritional Information: 257 Calories, 14g Protein, 46g Carbs, 7g Fat, 80mg sodium

Ingredients:
- 1½ c. water
- ½ c. steel cut oats
- 1/8 tsp. salt
- 1 c. whole wheat flour
- ½ tsp. baking powder
- ½ tsp. baking soda
- 1 egg
- 1 c. milk
- ½ c. Greek yogurt
- 1 c. frozen blueberries
- **¾ c. agave nectar**

Directions:
1. Combine your oats, salt, and water together in a medium saucepan, stir, and allow to come to a boil over high heat.
2. Lower heat, and allow to simmer for about 10 min, or until oats get tender. Set aside.
3. Combine all your remaining ingredients, except agave nectar, in a medium bowl then fold in oats.
4. Preheat your griddle, and lightly grease.
5. Cook ¼ cup of batter at a time for about 3 minutes per side.
6. Garnish with agave.

Spinach, Mushroom, And Feta Cheese Scramble

Preparation time: 3 mins

Servings: 1

Nutritional Information: 236.5 Calories, 22.2g Protein, 12.9g Carbs, 11.4g Fat, 502mg sodium.

Ingredients:
- olive oil cooking spray
- ½ c. sliced mushrooms
- 1 c. chopped spinach
- 3 eggs
- 2 tbsp. Feta cheese
- **pepper**

Directions:
1. Set a lightly greased, medium skillet over medium heat.
2. Add spinach, and mushrooms, and cook until spinach wilts.
3. Combine egg whites, cheese, pepper, and whole egg together in a medium bowl then whisk to combine.
4. Pour into your skillet and cook, while stirring, until set (about 4 minutes).
5. **Serve.**

Refrigerator Overnight Oatmeal

Preparation time: 5 mins

Servings: 2

Nutritional information: 244 Calories, 16g Protein, 37g Carbs, 5g Fat, 52mg sodium

Ingredients:
- 1c. oats
- 1 c. non-fat yogurt
- ½ c. milk
- 1 c. frozen blueberries
- **1 tbsp. Chia seeds**

Directions:
1. Add all your ingredients to a medium mixing bowl, and stir.
2. Split evenly among 2 airtight containers, seal, and refrigerate overnight.
3. **Serve.**

Red Velvet Pancakes With Cream Cheese Topping

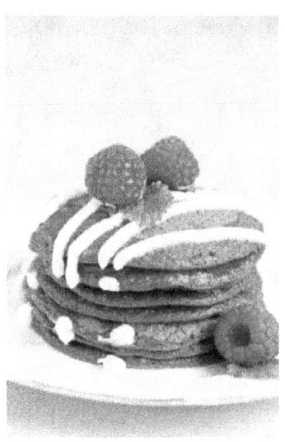

Preparation time: 15 mins

Servings: 2

Nutritional Information: 231 Calories, 7g Protein, 43g Carbs, 4g Fat, 560mg sodium

Ingredients:
Cream Cheese Topping:
- 2 oz. cream cheese
- 3 tbsp. yogurt
- 3 tbsp. honey
- **1 tbsp. milk**

Pancakes:
- ½ c. whole wheat flour
- ½ c. all-purpose flour
- 2¼ tsp. baking powder
- ½ tsp. unsweetened cocoa powder
- ¼ tsp. salt

- ¼ c. sugar
- 1 large egg
- 1 c. + 2 tbsp. milk
- 1 tsp. vanilla
- **1 tsp. red paste food coloring**

Directions:
1. Combine all your topping ingredients in a medium bowl, and set aside.
2. Add all your pancake ingredients together in a large bowl and fold until combined.
3. Set a greased skillet over medium heat to get hot.
4. Add ¼ cup of pancake batter onto the hot skillet and cook until bubbles begin to form on the top.
5. Flip and cook until set. Repeat until your batter is done.
6. **Add your toppings and serve.**

Peanut Butter & Banana Breakfast Smoothie

Preparation time: 2 mins

Servings: 1

Nutritional Information: 295 Calories, 133g Protein, 42g Carbs, 8.4g Fat, 308mg sodium

Ingredients:
- 1 c. non-fat milk
- 1 tbsp. peanut butter
- 1 banana
- **½ tsp. vanilla**

Directions:
1. Place, non-fat milk, peanut butter and banana in a blender.
2. **Blend until smooth.**

Mushroom Shallot Frittata

Preparation time: 3 mins

Servings: 4

Nutritional Information: 346 Calories, 19.1g Protein, 48.3g Carbs, 12g Fat, 217mg sodium

Ingredients:
- 1 tsp. butter
- 4 chopped shallots
- ½ lb. chopped mushrooms
- 2 tsps. chopped parsley
- 1 tsp. dried thyme
- black pepper
- 3 medium eggs
- 5 large egg whites
- 1 tbsp. milk
- **¼ c. grated parmesan cheese**

Directions:
1. Heat oven to 350 degrees.
2. In a suitable size oven-proof skillet, heat butter over medium flame.
3. Add shallots and sauté for about 5 mins. or until golden brown.
4. Add to pot, thyme, parsley, chopped mushroom and black pepper to taste.
5. Whisk milk, egg whites, parmesan and eggs into a bowl.
6. Pour mixture into the skillet ensuring the mushroom is totally covered.
7. Transfer the skillet to the oven as soon as the edges begin to set.
8. Bake until frittata is cooked (15-20 mins).
9. **Should be served warm, cut into equal wedges (4 pcs).**

Jack-O-Lantern Pancakes

Preparation time: 6 mins

Servings: 8

Nutritional Information: 313 Calories, 15g Protein, 28g Carbs, 16g Fat, 480mg sodium

Ingredients:
- 1 egg
- ½ c. canned pumpkin
- 1¾ c. low-fat milk
- 2 tbsp. vegetable oil
- 2 c. flour
- 2 tbsp. brown sugar
- 1 tbsp. baking powder
- 1 tsp. pumpkin pie spice
- **¼ tsp. salt**

Directions:
1. In a large mixing bowl, combine pumpkin, eggs, milk, and oil.
2. Add dry ingredients to egg mixture. Stir gently.
3. Coat griddle lightly with cooking spray and heat on medium.
4. When the griddle is hot, spoon (using a dessert spoon) batter onto griddle.
5. **When bubbles start bursting, flip pancakes over and cook until it's a nice golden-brown color.**

Morning Quinoa

Preparation time: 10 mins

Servings: 4

Nutritional Information: 287 Calories, 10.2g Protein, 52g Carbs, 5g Fat, 13mg sodium

Ingredients:
- 2 c. non-fat milk
- 1 c. quinoa
- ¼ c. brown sugar
- ½ tsp. cinnamon
- ¼ c. sliced slivered almonds
- **¼ c. dried currants**

Directions:
1. Wash the quinoa properly.
2. Bring the milk to a boil in a medium saucepan.
3. Add quinoa and continue boiling. Cover pot and bring flame to low and simmer until most of the liquid is dissolved (about 15 mins).
4. Turn off heat and use a fork to fluff. Add other ingredients and mix well.
5. **Cover and put aside for 15 mins.**

Fruit-N-Grain Breakfast Salad

Preparation time: 2 mins

Servings: 6

Nutritional Information: 116 Calories, 3g Protein, 24.5g Carbs, 1g Fat, 37mg sodium

Ingredients:
- 3 c. water
- ¼ tsp. salt
- ¾ c. brown rice
- ¾ c. bulgur
- 1 diced green apple
- 1 diced red apple
- 1 orange
- 1 c. raisins
- **8 oz. vanilla yogurt**

Directions:
1. Over high flame, boil water in a large pot.
2. Add the bulgur and the rice, lower flame. Close lid and allow cooking time of 10 mins.
3. After cooking, remove from heat, cover for 2 mins; set aside.
4. On a baking sheet, lay hot grains to cool (will give you a fluffier look). Can be prepared overnight and refrigerate.
5. Prepare fruit; core and dice your apples, just before serving. Peel and section your orange.
6. Remove chilled grains from refrigerator; transfer to a medium size mixing bowl, add cut fruit.
7. **Mix in yogurt into grains until well coated.**

Flax Banana Yogurt Muffins

Preparation time: 10 mins

Servings: 12

Nutritional Information: 136 Calories, 4g Protein, 30g Carbs, 2g Fat, 133mg sodium

Ingredients:
- 1 c. whole wheat flour
- 1 c. old-fashioned rolled oats
- 1 tsp. baking soda
- 2 tbsp. ground flaxseed
- 3 large ripe bananas
- ½ c. Greek yogurt
- ¼ c. unsweetened applesauce
- ¼ c. brown sugar
- **2 tsp. vanilla extract**

Directions:
1. Set oven at 355 degrees F and preheat.
2. Prepare muffin tin (can use cooking spray or cupcake liners.
3. Combine dry ingredients in a mixing bowl.
4. In a separate bowl, mix yogurt, banana, sugar, vanilla, and applesauce.
5. Combine both mixtures and mix. Do not over mix. Batter should not be smooth but lumpy.
6. **Bake for 20 mins. or when inserted toothpick comes out clean.**

Lunch Recipes

Veggie Quesadillas With Cilantro Yogurt Dip

Preparation time: 20 mins

Servings: 3

Nutritional Information: 344 Calories, 27g Protein, 46g Carbs, 8g Fat, 300mg sodium

Ingredients:
- 1 c. black beans
- 2 tbsp. chopped cilantro
- ½ chopped bell pepper
- ½ c. corn kernels
- 1 c. shredded cheese
- 6 corn tortillas
- 1 shredded carrot
- **½ minced jalapeno pepper**

Directions:
1. Set your skillet to preheat on low heat.
2. Lay 3 tortillas on a flat surface. Top evenly with peppers, carrots, cilantro, beans, corn, and cheese over the tortillas (covering each with another tortilla, maximum.
3. Add your quesadilla to your preheated skillet, and cook until the cheese melts, and tortilla becomes a nice golden brown (about 2 min).
4. **Flip to quesadilla, and cook for about a minute (or until golden).**

Mix well. Slice each quesadilla into 4 even wedges, and serve with your dip. Enjoy!

Sweet Roasted Beet & Arugula Tortilla Pizza

Preparation time: 10 mins

Servings: 6

Nutritional Information: 286 Calories, 15g Protein, 42g Carbs, 40g Fat, 265mg sodium

Ingredients:
- 2 chopped beets
- 6 corn tortillas
- 1 c. arugula
- ½ c. goat cheese
- 1 c. blackberries
- 2 tbsp. honey
- **2 tbsp. balsamic vinegar**

Directions:
1. Set your oven to preheat to 350 F.
2. Lay your tortillas on a flat surface. Top with beets, berries, and goat cheese.
3. Combine your balsamic vinegar, and honey together in a small bowl, and whisk to combine.
4. Drizzle the mixture over your pizza, and to bake for about 10 minutes, or until your cheese has melted slightly, and your tortilla crisp.
5. **Garnish with arugula, and serve.**

Pesto & Mozzarella Stuffed Portobello Mushroom Caps

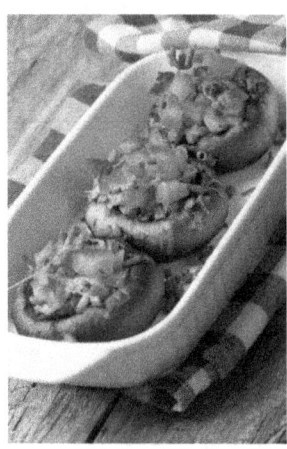

Preparation time: 15 mins

Servings: 2

Nutritional Information: 112 Calories:10.5g Protein, 7.5g Carbs, 5.4g Fat, 284mg sodium

Ingredients:
- 2 Portobello caps mushrooms
- 1 small diced tomato
- 2 tbsp. pesto
- **¼ c. shredded mozzarella cheese**

Directions:
1. Spoon your pesto evenly into your mushroom caps, then to with your remaining ingredients.
2. Set to bake at 400 degrees F for about 15 minutes.
3. **Enjoy!**

Southwestern Black Bean Cakes With Guacamole

Preparation time: 15 mins

Servings: 4

Nutritional Information: 178 Calories, 11g Protein, 25g Carbs, 7g Fat, 478mg sodium

Ingredients:
- 1 c. whole wheat bread crumbs
- 3 tbsp. chopped cilantro
- 2 garlic cloves
- 15 oz. black beans
- 7 oz. chipotle peppers in Adobo sauce
- 1 tsp. ground cumin
- 1 large egg
- ½ medium diced avocado
- 1 tbsp. lime juice
- **1 small tomato**

Directions:
1. Drain beans then add all your ingredients, except avocado, lime juice, and eggs, to a food processor and run until the mixture begin to pull away from the sides of processor.
2. Transfer to a large bowl, and add in egg then mix well.
3. Form into 4 even patties, and cook on a preheated, greased grill over medium heat for about 10 minutes, flipping halfway through.
4. Add your avocado, and lime juice in a small bowl, then stir and mash together using a fork.
5. **Season to taste then serve with bean cakes.**

Southwest Style Rice Bowl

Preparation time: 5 mins

Servings: 2

Nutritional Information: 168 Calories, 5.5g Protein, 18g Carbs, 8.2g Fat, 230mg sodium

Ingredients:
- 1 tbsp. vegetable oil
- 1 c. chopped vegetables
- 1 c. chopped chicken breast
- 1 c. brown rice
- 4 tbsp. salsa
- 2 tbsp. shredded cheddar cheese
- **2 tbsp. sour cream**

Directions:
1. Set a skillet with oil to heat up over medium heat.
2. Add chopped vegetables and allow to cook, while stirring, until vegetables become fork tender.
3. Add chicken, and brown rice and continue to cook, while stirring, until fully heated through.
4. **Split between 2 serving bowls, and garnish with your remaining ingredients. Serve, and enjoy!**

Pear, Turkey And Cheese Sandwich

Preparation time: 3 mins

Servings: 2

Nutritional Information: 337.3 Calories, 16.5g Protein, 55.8g Carbs, 11.6g Fat, 214mg sodium

Ingredients:
- 2 slices of bread
- 2 tsp. Dijon mustard
- 2 slices smoked turkey
- 1 sliced pear
- ¼ c. shredded mozzarella cheese
- **1/8 tsp. ground pepper**

Directions:
1. Use your mustard to spread on both slices of bread, then top each side with turkey and set one side aside.
2. Top your remaining half with pear slices, and season with pepper.
3. Close your sandwich, and set to broil for about 3 minutes, or until your cheese has been melted, and turkey warmed.
4. **Enjoy!**

Salmon Salad Pita

Preparation time: 5 mins

Servings: 3

Nutritional Information: 239 Calories, 25g Protein, 19g Carbs, 7g Fat, 440mg sodium

Ingredients:
- ¾ c. salmon
- 3 tbsp. yogurt
- 1 tbsp. lemon juice
- 2 tbsp. minced bell pepper
- 1 tbsp. minced red onion
- 1 tsp. chopped capers
- 1 tsp. dried dill
- 3 lettuce
- black pepper
- **3 whole wheat Pita bread**

Directions:
1. In a bowl, create your salmon salad by combining your first 8 ingredients, then stir.
2. Create salmon pita by spooning your salmon salad evenly onto your letter leaf then placing it inside your pitas.
3. **Enjoy!**

Fresh Shrimp Spring Rolls

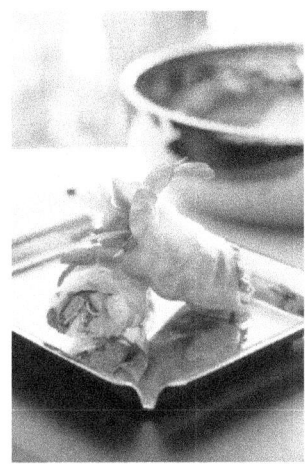

Preparation time: 20 mins

Servings: 12

Nutritional Information: 67 Calories, 2.62g Protein, 7.39g Carbs, 2.97g Fat, 290mg sodium

Ingredients:
- 12 sheets rice paper
- 12 leave bib lettuce
- 12 basil leaves
- ¾ c. cilantro
- 1 shredded carrot
- ½ sliced cucumber
- **200 oz. cooked shrimp**

Directions:
1. Add all your vegetables, and shrimp to separate bowls and lay out on a flat surface. Set a damp paper towel tower flat on your work surface.

2. Quickly wet one of your rice papers under warm water and lay on paper towel.
3. Top with 1 of each vegetable, and 4 pieces of shrimp, then roll your rice paper into a burrito – like roll.
4. Repeat until all your vegetables and shrimp has been used up.
5. **Serve, and enjoy.**

Sunshine Wrap

Preparation time: 20 mins

Servings: 4

Nutritional Information: 280.8 Calories, 19g Protein, 3g Carbs, 21.1g Fat, 148mg sodium

Ingredients:
- 8 oz. grilled chicken breast
- ½ c. diced celery
- 2/3 c. mandarin oranges
- ¼ c. minced onion
- 2 tbsp. mayonnaise
- 1 tp. soy sauce
- ¼ tsp. garlic powder
- ¼ tsp. black pepper
- 1 large whole wheat tortilla
- **4 lettuce leaves**

Directions:
1. Combine all your ingredients, except tortilla, and lettuce in a large bowl and toss to evenly coat.
2. Lay your tortillas down on a flat surface and cut into quarters.
3. **Top each quarter with a lettuce leaf, and spoon your chicken mixture into the middle of each.**

Roll each tortilla into a cone and seal by slightly wetting the edge with water. Enjoy!

Heartfelt Tuna Melt

Preparation time: 15 mins

Servings: 4

Nutritional Information: 197 Calories, 16g Protein, 21g Carbs, 6g Fat, 824mg sodium

Ingredients:
- 6 oz. white tuna packed in water
- 1/3 c. chopped celery
- ¼ c. chopped onion
- ¼ c. thousand island salad dressing
- 2 whole wheat English muffins
- 3 oz. grated cheddar cheese
- salt
- **black pepper**

Directions:
1. Heat broiler.
2. In a container, combine tuna, onion, celery and salad dressing.
3. Season to taste with salt and pepper.
4. Toast the halves of the English muffin.
5. On baking tray, place split side up, place 1/4 of tuna mixture on each half.
6. Broil for 3 mins or until heat is penetrated.
7. Place cheese on top and return tray to broiler for a minute longer or until cheese is melted.
8. **Serve, and enjoy.**

Apple-Swiss Panini

Preparation time: 8 mins

Servings: 4

Nutritional Information: 367 Calories, 24g Protein, 56g Carbs, 6g Fat, 84mg sodium

Ingredients:
- 8 slices whole-grain bread
- ¼ c. honey mustard
- 2 sliced apples
- 6 oz. sliced Swiss cheese
- 1 c. arugula leaves
- **cooking spray**

Directions:
1. On medium flame, preheat panini press on medium heat. Just use a non-stick skillet if you don't have a panini press.
2. Spread lightly, honey mustard evenly over each slice of bread.
3. Place layers of apple slices, arugula leaves, and cheese over 4 bread slices.
4. Use remaining bread slices to top each.
5. Coat panini press lightly with cooking spray.
6. Allow 3 to 5 mins to grill sandwiches or until cheese has melted and bread toasted.
7. **Transfer from pan and cool slightly before serving.**

California Grilled Veggie Sandwich

Preparation time: 15 mins

Servings: 4

Nutritional Information: 178 Calories, 6g Protein, 9g Carbs, 14g Fat, 223mg sodium

Ingredients:
- 3 tbsp. mayonnaise
- 3 minced garlic cloves
- 1 tbsp. lemon juice
- 1/8 c. olive oil
- 1 c. sliced red bell peppers
- 1 sliced zucchini
- 1 sliced red onion
- 1 sliced yellow squash
- 2 slices focaccia bread
- **½ c. Feta cheese**

Directions:
1. Mix in a small bowl, mayonnaise, minced garlic, and lemon juice.
2. Place in the refrigerator.
3. Heat grill for high heat.
4. Lightly grease both the grill and your vegetables.
5. Set zucchini and bell peppers closest to the middle of the grill; set squash and onion pieces around them.
6. Cook for 3 minutes on each side (total of 6 mins) transfer from grill and put aside briefly.
7. Coat cut sides of bread with mayonnaise mixture. Topped with sprinkled feta cheese. With cheese side up, place bread on the grill, and seal lid.
8. Grill for 2 to 3 minutes.
9. After bread is removed from grill, layer with vegetables.
10. Serve as open face sandwiches.

Chicken, Apple, And Spinach Salad

Preparation time: 10 mins

Servings: 4

Nutritional Information: 410 Calories, 30g Protein, 20g Carbs, 25g Fat, 786mg sodium

Ingredients
- 4 c. spinach
- 2 c. chopped apple
- 2 c. chopped chicken breast
- ½ c. sliced red onion
- ¼ c. chopped pecans
- **¾ c. Acai dressing**

Directions:
1. Set 4 salad bowls on the table and add spinach to each.
2. Add each of your remaining ingredients as layers on top of the greens.
3. **Once satisfied, drizzle each bowl of salad with 3 tablespoons of dressing.**

Coconut Shrimp

Preparation time: 10 mins

Servings: 4

Nutritional Information: 310 Calories, 9g Protein, 31g Carbs, 16g Fat, 560mg sodium

Ingredients:
- 1 lb. shrimp
- ¼ c. heavy cream
- 1 tbsp. lemon juice
- ¼ c. crushed chives
- 4 tbsp. butter
- 1 medium sliced tomato
- ¼ c. coconut water
- salt
- pepper
- **pecans**

Directions:
1. Melt butter in skillet over medium heat.
2. Place shrimp in pan and sauté for one minute.
3. Take off burner and pour in Coconut water and add back to burner.
4. Allow to cook for a few minutes while tossing then remove the shrimp and set aside.
5. Place heavy cream and tomatoes in a saucepan, bring the heat to a medium until thickened, pour in lemon juice and season with salt and pepper.
6. **Drop the shrimp back into the mixture and warm in sauce. Plate and sprinkle chives and pecans.**

Steamed Spinach

Preparation time: 10 mins

Servings: 1

Nutritional Information: 74 Calories, 5. 33g Protein, 6.81g Carbs, 4.16g Fat, 126mg sodium

Ingredients:
- 1tsp. salt
- 2 oz. vegetable oil
- 2 oz. onion
- 1 tsp. scotch bonnet pepper
- 4 oz. sliced carrot
- 1 bundle spinach
- 1 tsp. black pepper
- 4 oz. tomato
- 1 oz. green onion
- 1 tsp. thyme
- **1 tsp. unsalted butter**

Directions:
1. Add your oil, carrots, pepper, and onions to a skillet and sauté until soft (for about a minute).
2. Add Spinach to skillet and season with salt and pepper to taste.
3. Cover and allow to cook for another 3 minutes.
4. **Add your remaining ingredients to your pot allow to cook until spinach is tender (about 3 minutes longer).**

Cinnamon Sweet Potatoes

Preparation time: 10 mins

Servings: 3

Nutritional Information: 145.3 Calories, 1.7g Protein, 35.2g Carbs, 0.4g Fat, 14mg sodium

Ingredients:
- 3 sweet potatoes
- ½ tsp. cinnamon powder
- 1 sliced onion
- ½ tsp. black pepper
- ¼ tsp. salt
- **2 tbsp. olive oil**

Directions:
1. Heat oil in pan and sauté onion for 1-2 minutes. Set aside.
2. Now combine sweet potatoes with onion and season with salt, pepper and cinnamon powder.
3. Preheat oven at 355 degrees.
4. **Transfer to serving dish and bake for 30-35 minutes.**

Chicken Santa Fe

Preparation time: 5 mins

Servings: 2

Nutritional Information: 370 Calories, 30g Protein, 29g Carbs, 15g Fat, 540mg sodium

Ingredients:
- 15 oz. canned corn
- 6 chicken breasts
- 15 oz. canned black beans
- 1 c. shredded cheddar cheese
- **1 c. salsa**

Directions:
1. Set slow cooker on high.
2. Combine corn, half of salsa and beans in slow cooker.
3. Put in chicken and top with remaining salsa.
4. Cover pot and cook for 2 hours 55 min or until chicken is thoroughly cooked.
5. **Top with cheese and cook for 5 mins more or until cheese melts.**

Kung Pao Shrimp

Preparation time: 15 mins

Servings: 2

Nutritional Information: 346 Calories, 14g Protein, 34g Carbs, 19g Fat, 950mg sodium

Ingredients:
- 2 tbsp. oil
- 1 sliced ginger
- ¼ c. onion
- 10 red chilies
- 12 oz. shrimp
- ¼ c. roasted peanuts
- 3 scallion stalks
- Kung Pao sauce
- 2 tbsp. soy sauce
- 2 tbsp. sweet soy sauce
- ½ tsp. cornstarch
- 4 tbsp. water
- ½ tsp. sesame oil
- ¼ tsp. white pepper
- ½ tsp. apple cider vinegar
- **½ tsp. sugar**

Directions:
1. Mix ingredients for sauce together and put aside till needed.
2. Heat oil in a wok then add ginger and stir. Put in green pepper, onion, and chilies.
3. Until you smell the chilies then add peanuts and shrimp and stir.
4. Add Kung Pao when shrimp has almost cooked.
5. **Stir frequently to avoid sticking. Cook until sauce thickens then add scallions. Remove from heat and serve hot.**

Banana Waffles

Preparation time: 10 mins

Servings: 6

Nutritional Information: 197.5 Calories, 7.9g Protein, 37.9g Carbs, 3.1g Fat, 491mg sodium

Ingredients:
- 3 eggs
- 1 c. all-purpose flour
- 3 tbsp. melted butter
- 1 c. whole-wheat flour
- 1 ½ c. milk
- 2 tsp. baking powder
- ¼ tsp. salt
- 2 tbsp. honey
- **2 ripe bananas**

Directions:
1. In a bowl combine the flours, salt and baking powder.
2. In a blender combine the milk, honey, melted butter, and bananas.
3. Process until smooth.
4. Fold the banana mix into the dry ingredients and continue stirring until smooth. Let the batter rest for 10 minutes and preheat the waffle iron.
5. Pour 1/3 cup batter on the iron and cook for 4 minutes.
6. **Serve with fresh fruits.**

Bbq Baked Beans

Preparation time: 10 mins

Servings: 3

Nutritional Information: 210 Calories, 8g Protein, 41g Carbs, 1.5g Fat, 780mg sodium

Ingredients:
- 1 chopped yellow onion
- 5 minced garlic cloves
- 1 chopped jalapeno
- ¼ lb. diced potatoes
- 1 lb. pinto
- 6 c. water
- 1 c. BBQ sauce
- ½ c. dark brown sugar
- 2 tbsp. spicy brown mustard
- 2 tbsp. Adobe sauce
- 2 tbsp. Tabasco sauce
- 2 tsp. salt
- **2 tsp. pepper**

Directions:
1. Set your Dutch oven to preheat on the top of the stove.
2. Add potatoes to the heated oven and allow to brown. At this point, add the jalapeno and onions then proceed to sauté until onions become soft.
3. Continue to sauté while you add the garlic. Continue for about a minute.
4. Pour in the beans, and water then cover and allow cooking on low to medium heat for about an hour or until the beans become soft.
5. Add a bit of your preferred BBQ sauce along with the brown sugar, adobo sauce, Tabasco, mustard salt and pepper while stirring well.

6. Remove the cover and allow simmering until the sauce thickens and the beans become completely cooked.

Dinner Recipes

Beef Stew With Fennel And Shallots

Preparation time: 10 mins

Servings: 6

Nutritional Information: 244 calories, 8g fat, 22g carbs, 21g protein, 185mg sodium

Ingredients:
- 1/3 c. chopped fresh parsley
- 3 Portobello mushrooms
- 18 small boiling onions
- 4 large red-skinned potatoes
- 4 large sliced carrots
- 3 c. vegetable stock
- 1 bay leaf
- 2 fresh thyme sprigs
- ¾ tsp. ground black pepper
- 3 large shallots
- ½ fennel bulb
- 2 tbsp. olive oil
- 1 lb. boneless lean beef stew meat
- **3 tbsp. all- purpose flour**

Directions:
1. Start by placing the flour on a place and rolling the beef cubes in the flour
2. Then, using a large saucepan, pour the oil in and heat at medium heat.
3. Once the beef is floured, put it into the saucepan and cook until brown on all sides.
4. Remove the beef and let cook elsewhere.
5. Without changing the temperature, place the shallots and the fennel in the pan and cook until they are a light brown.

6. Add the lay leaf, thyme sprigs, and a quarter of the pepper to the mix and let cook for a minute or two.
7. Now, add the beef back into the pan with the vegetable stock and bring the mixture to a boil. After, reduce the heat and cover it while it simmers. Leave it like this for 45 minutes.
8. Once the meat is tender, add the mushrooms, onions, potatoes, and carrots.
9. Stir the mixture and let simmer for another 30 minutes.
10. Pull the bay leaf and the thyme sprigs out of the stew and stir in the parsley and remaining pepper.
    Serve immediately.

Grilled Portobello Mushroom Burger

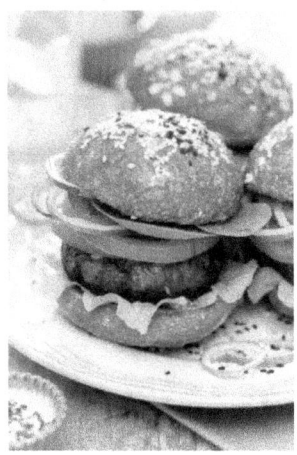

Preparation time: 15 mins

Servings: 4

Nutritional Information: 301 calories, 9g fat, 45g carbs, 10g protein, 163mg sodium

Ingredients:
- 2 romaine lettuce leaves
- 4 slices of red onion
- 1 slices of tomato
- 4 whole-wheat toasted buns
- 2 tbsp. olive oil
- ¼ tsp. cayenne pepper
- 1 minced garlic clove
- 1 tbsp. sugar
- ½ c. water
- 1/3 c. balsamic vinegar
- **4 large Portobello mushroom caps**

Directions:

1. The Portobello mushrooms need to be cleaned and their stems need to be removed and the caps need to be set aside.
2. Now, in a small bowl the olive oil, cayenne pepper, garlic, sugar, water, and vinegar need to be mixed together and pored over top the mushroom caps.
3. The caps need to be placed into a plastic container, covered, and placed into the refrigerator to marinate for an hour.
4. Turn on the grill and lightly coat it in cooking spray—or, turn on the stove and coat a frying pan in the same substance.
5. Fry or grill the mushrooms on medium heat, making sure to flip them often. Usually, it will take five minutes on each side.
6. Place the mushrooms on their own bun and top with half a lettuce leaf, one onion slice and one tomato slice.
7. **Serve immediately.**

Chicken Brats

Preparation time: 10 mins

Servings: 6

Nutritional Information: 156 calories, 4g fat, 12g carbs, 18g protein, 92mg sodium

Ingredients:
- 1 tsp. celery seed
- 1 tsp. ground mustard seed
- ¼ tsp. nutmeg
- 1 tsp. minced rosemary
- ½ tsp. cayenne pepper
- ½ tsp. white pepper
- 1 tsp. black pepper
- 1 tsp. paprika
- 1 tsp. cumin seed
- 2 tsp. fennel seed
- 1 lb. ground chicken breast
- 1 c. cooked brown rice
- ½ tsp. canola oil
- 4 minced garlic
- **1 c. minced yellow onion**

Ingredients:
1. In a frying pan, sauté the canola oil, garlic, and onion until golden.
2. Place the browned onion and garlic in the cooked rice and mix in all the other herbs and spices with the ground chicken breast.
3. Let the mixture marinate in the fridge for about an hour.
4. Pre-heat the oven to 350 degrees Fahrenheit.
5. Remove from the fridge and roll the mixture into sausage shapes and place on a cooking sheet.
6. Bake in the oven for about 5-10 minutes, or until cooked.

7. Let the sausages cool before serving.

Asian Pork Tenderloin

Preparation time: 20 mins

Servings: 4

Nutritional Information: 248 calories, 1g carbs, 16g fat, 26g protein, 57mg sodium

Ingredients:
- 1 lb. pork tenderloin
- 1 tbsp. sesame seed oil
- 1/8 tsp. ground cinnamon
- ¼ tsp. ground cumin
- ½ tsp. celery seed
- 1/8 tsp. cayenne pepper
- 1 tsp. ground coriander
- **2 tbsp. sesame seeds**

Directions:
1. Preheat the oven to 400 degrees Fahrenheit.
2. While the oven is preheating, grease a baking sheet with cooking spray.
3. Pull out a frying pan and on low heat fry the sesame seeds while stirring contently.
4. After one to two minutes, or the sesame seeds are golden brown, remove the seeds from the heat and set them aside.
5. In a large mixing bowl, place the toasted sesame seeds, sesame seed oil, cinnamon, cumin, celery seed, cayenne pepper, and coriander inside and stir until it is mixed evenly.
6. Using the prepared baking dish, place the tenderloin on top and evenly space them out.
7. Use a brush to lather the tenderloin, on both sides, with the mixture.

8. Place the baking sheet inside the oven and let bake for about 15 minutes or until they are no longer pink. Take the tenderloin out and serve with a side dish immediately.

White Chicken Chili

Preparation time: 10 mins

Servings: 8

Nutritional Information: 212 calories, 4g fat, 25g carbs, 19g protein, 241g sodium

Ingredients:
- 3 tbsp. chopped cilantro
- 8 tbsp. shredded Monterey jack cheese
- 1 tsp. cayenne pepper
- 1 tsp. dried oregano
- 1 tsp. ground cumin
- 2 tsp. chili powder
- 2 minced garlic cloves
- 1 sliced red pepper
- ½ sliced green pepper
- 4 c. low-sodium chicken broth
- 1 can diced tomatoes
- 2 cans white beans
- **1 can white chunk chicken**

Directions:
1. Grab a large cooking pot and place the chicken broth, tomatoes, and chicken inside.
2. Bring the mixture to a boil and then cover it to let it simmer.
3. While the mixture is simmering, take a non-stick frying pan, cover it in cooking spray, and add the garlic, peppers, and onions.
4. Fry the vegetables until golden brown or to your liking.
5. Add the contents of the frying pan to the cooking pot.
6. Add the cayenne pepper, oregano, cumin, and chili powder and cover the mixture again.

7. Raise the heat up to medium and let it simmer for about ten more minutes.
8. Ladle the chili into bowls and serve immediately.
9. **Use cilantro only as a garnish.**

Saucy Chicken

Preparation time: 15 mins

Servings: 4

Nutritional Information: 125.5 Calories, 11.7g Protein, 16.7g Carbs, 1.6g Fat, 791mg sodium

Ingredients:
- 8 chicken tights
- 1 c. chicken broth
- 1 tbsp. sherry vinegar
- 1½ c. roasted red peppers, chopped
- 4 crushed garlic cloves
- 1½ c. diced russet potatoes
- **2 tsp. chopped thyme leaves**

Directions:
1. Preheat oven to 425F.
2. Heat olive oil in a pan over medium-high heat.
3. Season the chicken tights with salt and pepper and place into heated oil, skin side down. Cook the chicken without moving around for 3 minutes or until browned. Transfer to a plate and repeat with remaining chicken.
4. Add the garlic and thyme to the same skillet. Cook until fragrant.
5. Add the potatoes, chicken broth, red peppers, and vinegar to the pan.
6. Bring to boil and once boils remove from the heat.
7. Return the chicken to the pan, skin side up and place in the oven.
8. Braise the chicken for 30 minutes or until the potatoes are tender.
9. **Serve while still hot with baguette or some other bread.**

Baked Salmon

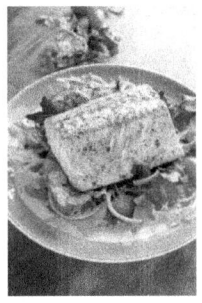

Preparation time: 10 mins

Servings: 6

Nutritional Information: 274 Calories, 24g Protein, 1g Carbs, 19g Fat, 284mg sodium

Ingredients:
- 1½ lbs. salmon fillets
- ½ sliced onion
- 1 c. chopped grape tomatoes
- 1 tsp. dried basil
- 1 tbsp. chopped chives
- 1 tsp. dried rosemary
- 1 tsp. garlic powder
- 1 tsp. salt
- 1/3 c. soy sauce
- 1/3 c. brown sugar
- 1/3 c. water
- **¼ c. vegetable oil**

Directions:
1. Preheat oven to 350 degrees.
2. Season salmon fillets with onion, basil, rosemary, garlic powder, and salt.

3. In a small bowl, combine brown sugar, soy sauce, water, and vegetable oil until sugar is dissolved.
4. Place fillets in a Ziploc bag or airtight container with soy sauce mixture and allow to marinate in the refrigerator for at least 2 hours.
5. **Preheat grill at medium heat. Lightly oil grill grate. Place fillets on the preheated grill and cook for 6 to 8 minutes per side.**

Roasted Turkey

Preparation time: 15 mins

Servings: 6

Nutritional Information: 240.4 Calories, 3.7g Protein, 47.4g Carbs, 4.3g Fat, 71mg sodium

Ingredients:
- 1 whole turkey
- 2 tsp. garlic paste
- 1 tsp. ginger powder
- 2 tablespoons soya sauce
- 1 tsp. cayenne pepper
- 1 tsp. salt
- ½ tsp. black pepper
- 3 tbsp. lemon juice
- 2 tbsp. red wine vinegar
- ½ tsp. mustard powder
- 1 tsp. cinnamon powder
- **2 tbsp. sesame seeds oil**

Directions:
1. In a bowl add garlic paste, ginger powder, cayenne pepper, black pepper, cinnamon powder, mustard powder, lemon juice, oil, vinegar, soya sauce and salt, mix well.
2. Now pour this marinate over turkey and rub with hands all over it.
3. Cover and leave to marinade for 15-20 minutes. Preheat oven at 355 degrees.
4. Spread aluminum foil in baking tray and place turkey on it.
5. Bake for 40-45 minutes or till nicely golden.
6. **Serve and enjoy.**

Chicken Fried Rice

Preparation time: 6 mins

Servings: 2

Nutritional Information: 309.6 Calories, 15g Protein, 50g Carbs, 5g Fat, 869mg sodium

Ingredients:
- 2 tbsp. oil
- 2 minced garlic cloves
- 4 oz. cubed chicken breast
- 4 oz. shrimps
- 1 c. mix vegetables-frozen
- 12 oz. overnight rice
- 1 tbsp. fish sauce
- 1 tbsp. soy sauce
- ¼ tsp. oyster sauce
- ¼ tsp. white pepper
- 2 eggs
- **¼ tsp. salt**

Directions:
1. Put oil in a pan and add garlic, cook, until the aroma of the garlic becomes present.
2. Add shrimp, chicken, and vegetables.
3. Put in rice and stir to combine with veggies.
4. Add soy sauce, fish sauce, oyster sauce, salt, and pepper and stir the rice for a few minutes.
5. Use a spatula to make a gap in the center of the rice.
6. Dispense eggs in the center and let it sit for 30 seconds.
7. Use rice to cover eggs and stir as egg cooks.
8. **Add some salt and stir a bit more then serve.**

Buffalo & Ranch Chicken Meatloaf

Preparation time: 10 mins

Servings: 6

Nutritional Information: 119 Calories, 6g Protein, 14g Carbs, 4g Fat, 880mg sodium

Ingredients:
- ½ c. Ranch dressing
- ¼ c. Buffalo wing sauce
- 675g ground chicken
- 120g chicken stuffing mix
- ½ c. Feta cheese
- 1 sliced celery stalk
- 2 chopped green onion
- **1 egg**

Directions:
1. Set your oven to preheat to 375 degrees and lightly grease a 6 x 4-inch loaf tin with olive oil.
2. Mix all your egg and dry ingredients, along with half of your dressing ingredients together until fully incorporated using your hands.
3. Once combined, add your meat mixture into your greased loaf tin, top with the other half of your dressing ingredients and set to bake until done (about 30 to 35 minutes).
4. **Tip: Use a thermometer to determine doneness by inserting it into the thickest part of the meatloaf. The temperature should be at least 165 degrees F.**

Shitake & Snow Peas Quinoa

Preparation time: 10 mins

Servings: 4

Nutritional Information:210 Calories, 8g Protein, 32g Carbs, 6g Fat, 321mg sodium

Ingredients:
- 3 c. fluffy quinoa
- 1 tbsp. sesame oil
- 1 tbsp. garlic cloves
- 4 oz. Shitake mushrooms
- 4 oz. snow peas
- ¼ tsp. salt
- ¼ tsp. pepper
- 1 tbsp. soy sauce
- **1 sliced green onion**

Directions:
1. In a medium non-stick skillet heat your sesame oil on medium heat.
2. Add your garlic and allow to cook for about a minute stirring frequently so that it doesn't burn.
3. Add in your mushrooms and cook until tender (should be about 5 min)
4. Next, add the snow peas, salt, and pepper. Then continue stirring until peas become bright green in color (it generally takes about 3 minutes) then remove from the heat.
5. Now, add in all the remaining ingredients and toss until fully combined.
6. **Serve and enjoy.**

Steamed Mussels

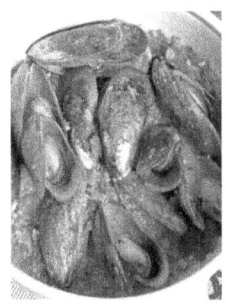

Preparation time: 5 mins

Servings: 4

Nutritional Information: 256 Calories, 35.4g Protein, 10.98g Carbs, 6.66g Fat, 90mg sodium

Ingredients:
- 6 oz. chorizo
- 1 c. white wine
- 2 tbsp. olive oil
- 1 sliced onion
- 4 lbs. mussels
- 3 sprigs thyme
- 1 tsp. smoked paprika
- 14.5 oz. diced tomatoes
- 4 sliced garlic cloves
- salt
- **pepper**

Directions:
1. Heat olive oil over medium-high heat until simmering.

2. Add the onion, season to taste and cook until softened for 3-4 minutes.
3. Add the garlic and cook for 1 minute more.
4. Stir in the smoked paprika and cook for 30 seconds or until fragrant.
5. Add the chorizo, wine, and tomatoes.
6. Add the fresh thyme and bring to a simmer.
7. Stir in the mussels and coat with sauce.
8. Cover and cook until mussels are opened.
9. **Discard all unopened ones.**

Serve mussels while still hot with toasted bread slices.

Gruyere And Spinach Casserole

Preparation time: 10 mins

Servings: 5

Nutritional Information: 270 Calories, 18g Protein, 8g Carbs, 19g Fat,165mg sodium

Ingredients:
- 2 c. chopped spinach
- 2 eggs
- 1 tsp. sugar
- 2 oz. grated gruyere
- 1 c. grated parmesan cheese
- ¼ tsp. salt
- ½ c. chopped green onion
- 4 minced garlic cloves
- 2 eggs
- 1 tsp. chili powder
- 1 c. heavy milk
- **2 tbsp. olive oil**

Directions:
1. Heat oil in saucepan and sauté garlic for 1 minute with onion.
2. Add spinach and stir for 2-3 minutes till its color is lightly changed.
3. In separate bowl add eggs and whisks for 1-2 minutes. Add in milk, gruyere and whisk again for 1 minute.
4. Transfer this mixture in spinach mixture and cook for 2 minutes.
5. Season with salt and chili powder.
6. Preheat oven at 355 degrees. Add gruyere mixture in baking dish, top with parmesan cheese and bake for 40-45 minutes.
7. **Serve and enjoy.**

Honey Garlic Chicken Drumsticks

Preparation time: 15 mins

Servings: 6

Nutritional Information: 121.2 Calories, 8.1g Protein, 15.5g Carbs, 3.3g Fat, 416mg sodium

Ingredients:
- 8 chicken drumsticks
- 3 tsp. garlic powder
- 1 tsp. ginger powder
- 3 tbsp. soya sauce
- 1 tsp. cayenne pepper
- 1 tsp. salt
- 2 tbsp. barbeque sauce
- 2 tbsp. lime juice
- ¼ c. apple cider vinegar
- 2 tbsp. olive oil
- **3 tbsp. honey**

Directions:
1. In a bowl add ginger powder, garlic powder, soya sauce, honey, vinegar, lime juice, barbeque sauce, salt, pepper and toss to combine.
2. Add in chicken drumsticks and mix well, leave to marinade for 20 minutes. Preheat oven at 355 degrees.
3. Transfer drumsticks in baking tray and bake for 30-35 minutes or till golden brown.
4. **Serve and enjoy.**

Shrimp Pasta Primavera

Preparation time: 15 mins

Servings: 6

Nutritional Information: 440 Calories, 31g Protein: 31g Carbs, 18g Fat, 420mg sodium

Ingredients:
- 1¼ c. sliced asparagus
- 12 oz. whole wheat penne
- 1 c. green peas
- 2 tsp. olive oil
- 1 tbsp. minced garlic
- 1/8 tsp. crushed red pepper
- 1 lb. shrimps
- ½ c. sliced green onion
- 2 tsp. lemon juice
- 1 tbsp. chopped parsley
- 1/3 c. grated parmesan cheese
- ½ tsp. salt
- **½ tsp. pepper**

Directions:
1. Set a large saucepan with water over high heat, and allow to come to a boil.
2. Once boiling, add asparagus then cook until fork tender (about 4 minutes). Carefully remove the asparagus from the hot water using a slotted spoon then add your pasta to the same pot.
3. Cook until done based on the instructions on the package. When the pasta was 2 minutes out add peas.
4. When fully cooked, drain, and add to a large bowl with the asparagus. Next, set a skillet with olive oil over medium heat, then add red pepper, and garlic, then cook, while stirring for about a minute.

5. Add shrimp and cook until it becomes opaque (about 4 minutes, stirring).
6. **Add your remaining ingredients to the skillet on top of shrimp and toss to coat.**

Salads & Soups Recipes

Easy Shrimp Salad

Preparation time: 10 mins

Servings: 6

Nutritional Information: 210 calories, 28g carbs, 14g protein, 255mg sodium

Ingredients:
For the shrimps:
- 2 minced garlic cloves
- 1 lb. shrimps
- 1 tsp. Cajun spice
- **2 tbsp. olive oil**

For the salad:
- 6 c. lettuce leaves
- 4 chopped tomatoes
- 1 chopped yellow onion
- 1 sliced cucumber
- 2 chopped avocados
- 1 c. corn
- 1 lemon
- ½ bunch chopped parsley
- 2 tbsp. olive oil
- **black pepper**

Directions:
1. In a bowl, combine the shrimp with Cajun spice and garlic and toss.
2. Heat up a pan with 2 tablespoons oil over medium-high heat, add shrimp, cook for 2 minutes on each side and transfer to a bowl.
3. Add lettuce, tomatoes, onion, cucumber, avocado, corn and a pinch of pepper and toss.

4. In a small bowl, mix 2 tablespoons oil with parsley and lemon juice, whisk well, pour over the salad, toss and serve.

Greek Chicken Salad

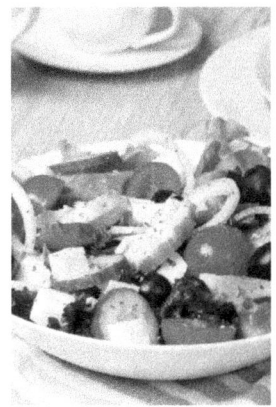

Preparation time: 10 minutes

Servings: 4

Nutritional Information: 180 calories, 10g fat, 16g carbs, 10g protein, 149mg sodium

Ingredients:
- 15 oz. canned chickpeas
- 9 oz. chicken breast
- 1 chopped cucumber
- 4 chopped green onions
- black pepper
- ½ c. yogurt
- ¼ c. chopped mint
- 2 c. baby spinach
- 2 minced garlic cloves
- 1/3 c. feta cheese
- **4 lemon wedges**

Directions:

1. In a salad bowl, mix chicken meat with chickpeas, cucumber, onions, mint, garlic, salt and pepper.
2. Add yogurt, spinach and feta and toss to coat.
3. Serve with lemon wedges on the side.
4. **Enjoy!**

Chicken Soup

Preparation time: 10 mins

Servings: 6

Nutritional Information: 200 calories, 10g fat, 16g carbs, 12g protein, 110mg sodium

Ingredients:
- 1 whole chicken
- 6 chopped celery stalks
- 6 sliced carrots
- 1 onion
- 1 bunch parsley springs
- 1 bunch dill springs
- 2 tbsp. chopped dill
- 3 garlic cloves
- 2 tbsp. black peppercorns
- black pepper
- 2 bay leaves
- **¼ tsp. saffron threads**

Directions:
1. Put chicken pieces in a pot, add water to cover, bring to a boil over medium-high heat, cook for 15 minutes and skim foam.
2. Add celery, onion, carrots, parsley springs, dill springs, whole cloves, bay leaves, peppercorns and some black pepper, stir, cover pot, reduce heat to medium-low and simmer for 1 hour and 30 minutes.
3. Take chicken pieces out and leave them aside to cool down.
4. Strain soup into another pot, reserve carrots and celery but discard herbs and spices.
5. Discard bones from the chicken, cut meat into strips and return to pot.
6. Heat up the soup with reserved veggies, add chicken pieces, crushed saffron and chopped dill and stir.

7. **Ladle soup into bowls and serve. Enjoy!**

Pumpkin Soup

Preparation time: 10 mins

Servings: 4

Nutritional Information: 180 calories, 10g fat, 22g carbs, 14g protein, 106mg sodium

Ingredients:
- 1 chopped yellow onion
- ¾ c. water
- 15 oz. pumpkin puree
- 2 c. veggie stock
- ½ tsp. cinnamon powder
- ¼ tsp. ground nutmeg
- 1 c. fat-free milk
- black pepper
- **1 chopped green onion**

Directions:
1. Put the water in a pot, bring to a simmer over medium heat, add onion, stock and pumpkin puree and stir.
2. Add cinnamon, nutmeg, milk and black pepper, stir, cook for 10 minutes, ladle into bowls, sprinkle green onion on top and serve.
3. **Enjoy!**

Spicy Black Bean Soup

Preparation time: 10 mins

Servings: 8

Nutritional Information: calories 220, fat 10, carbs 34, protein 14, 290mg sodium

Ingredients:
- 1 lb. black beans
- 2 chopped yellow onions
- 2 quarts low-sodium veggie stock
- 2 tbsp. olive oil
- 6 minced garlic cloves
- 2 chopped tomatoes
- 2 chopped jalapenos
- ½ tsp. dried oregano
- 1 tsp. ground cumin
- 1 tsp. grated ginger
- 2 bay leaves
- 1 tbsp. chili powder
- 3 tbsp. balsamic vinegar
- black pepper
- **½ c. chopped scallions**

Directions:
1. Put the stock in a pot, bring to a simmer over medium heat, add beans, cover and cook for 45 minutes.
2. Meanwhile, heat up a pan with the oil over medium-high heat, add ginger, garlic and onion, stir and cook for 5 minutes.
3. Add tomatoes, cumin, jalapeno, oregano and chili powder, stir, cook for 3 minutes more and transfer to the pot with the beans.
4. Add bay leaves, cover the pot and cook the soup for 40 minutes more.

5. Add vinegar, stir, cook the soup for 15 minutes more, discard bay leaves, blend the soup using an immersion blender, ladle into bowls and serve with scallions on top. Enjoy!

Shrimp Soup

Preparation time: 10 mins

Servings: 6

Nutritional Information: 190 calories, 8g fat, 30g carbs, 6g protein, 403mg sodium

Ingredients:
- 8 oz. shrimps
- 1 stalk lemongrass
- 2 grated ginger
- 6 c. low-sodium chicken stock
- 2 chopped jalapenos
- 4 lime leaves
- 1½ c. chopped pineapple
- 1 c. chopped shiitake mushroom caps
- 1 chopped tomato
- ½ cubed bell pepper
- 1 tsp. stevia
- ¼ c. lime juice
- 1/3 c. chopped cilantro
- **2 sliced scallions**

Directions:
1. In a pot, mix ginger with lemongrass, stock, jalapenos and lime leaves, stir, bring to a boil over medium heat, cover, cook for 15 minutes, strain liquid in a bowl and discard solids.
2. Return soup to the pot again, add pineapple, tomato, mushrooms, bell pepper, sugar and fish sauce, stir, bring to a boil over medium heat, cook for 5 minutes, add shrimp and cook for 3 more minutes.
3. **Add lime juice, cilantro and scallions, stir, ladle into soup bowls and serve.**

Enjoy!

Kale Salad With Mixed Vegetables

Preparation time: 10 mins

Servings: 4

Nutritional Information: 240 Calories, 9g Protein, 36g Carbs, 9g Fat, 192mg sodium

Ingredients:
- 1 bunch chopped Premier kale
- 1 c. fresh peas
- 2 chopped carrots
- 1 c. boiled potatoes
- 1 c. sliced cabbage
- 2 tbsp. apple cider vinegar
- 1 tsp. chili powder
- ½ tsp. salt
- 2 tbsp. coconut oil
- **1 tsp. coconut powder**

Directions:
1. Combine all vegetables with kale.
2. Drizzle vinegar and coconut oil.
3. Season with salt and chili powder.
4. Sprinkle coconut powder and toss to combine.
5. **Add to a serving dish and serve. Enjoy.**

Cream Of Corn Soup

Preparation time: 15 mins

Servings: 4

Nutritional Information: 223 Calories, 7.84g Protein, 23.98g Carbs, 11.51g Fat, 705mg sodium

Ingredients:
- 0.5 lb. corn puree
- 0.5 lb. carrots
- 2 c. vegetable stock
- ½ c. chopped onion
- ½ tsp. salt
- ¼ tsp. pepper
- 1 tsp. dried thyme
- 2 oz. chopped celery
- ½ tbsp. olive oil
- **1 anise star**

Directions:
1. Heat olive oil in medium pot and add onion; add celery, carrots and sauté for 15 minutes, until onion is caramelized.
2. Add corn and stir until corn is tender.
3. Add thyme and stir well.
4. Transfer the vegetables in a blender, add pumpkin puree, vegetable stock, and pulse until smooth.
5. Transfer the mixture into sauce pan and simmer, add anise star and simmer over medium-high heat for 5-8 minutes or until heated through.
6. Remove the anise star and discard.
7. **Serve immediately.**

Clam Soup

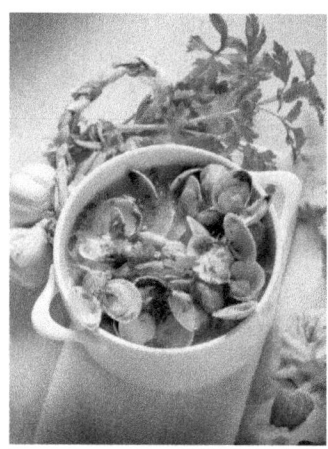

Preparation time: 15 mins

Servings: 4

Nutritional Information:80 Calories, 3g Protein, 16g Carbs, 0.5g Fat, 480mg sodium

Ingredients:
- 1½ c. water
- ½ fresh ginger
- 1 lb. Manila clams
- 1 tbsp. Chinese rice white wine
- ¼ tsp. salt
- **¼ tsp. white pepper**

Directions:
1. Boil water in a large pot and add clams and ginger.
2. Cook until clams open then add wine.
3. **Add pepper and salt and serve hot.**

Curried Quinoa Sweet Potato Salad

Preparation time: 12 mins

Servings: 6

Nutritional Information: 335.3 Calories, 5.5g Protein, 55.2g Carbs, 9g Fat, 30mg sodium

Ingredients:
- 1 c. curried quinoa
- 6 chopped sweet potatoes
- 1 c. water
- ¼ c. chopped onion
- 1 chopped celery
- salt
- pepper
- 3 boiled eggs
- 1 tbsp. chopped dill
- ½ c. mayonnaise
- 1 tsp. yellow mustard
- **1 tsp. vinegar**

Directions:
1. Pour in your potatoes and water into the cooker.
2. Securely close the lid and allow to rise to high pressure over a high flame. Cook for about 3 minutes.
3. Remove the cooker from the flame and cool under cold running water.
4. Proceed to peel and dice potatoes then layer them alternately with celery and onion.
5. Season with salt and pepper then add your dill and chopped eggs.
6. In a separate bowl combine the mustard, mayonnaise, and vinegar then fold the mixture gently into the potatoes.

7. Stir in your cooked quinoa.
8. **Chill, serve and enjoy!**

Desserts Recipes

Carrot Cupcakes

Preparation time: 15 mins

Servings: 6

Nutritional Information: 150 calories, 4g fat, 16g carbs, 8g protein, 190mg sodium

Ingredients:
- 1 c. almonds
- 2 c. carrot pulp
- 1 c. chopped dates
- ½ tsp. grated ginger
- 1 tsp. cinnamon powder
- 1 tsp. nutmeg
- **¾ c. raisins**

For the frosting:
- 1 c. cashews
- 1 tbsp. water
- 1 tsp. lemon juice
- **6 dates**

Directions:
1. In your food processor, mix 1 cup walnuts with 1 cup dates, carrot pulp, 1 teaspoon cinnamon, ginger, a pinch of nutmeg and the raisins, blend and divide this into cupcake cups.
2. Clean your food processor, add 1 cup cashews, 6 dates, a splash of water and the lemon juice and blend these as well.

3. Divide the frosting on the cupcakes, introduce them in the fridge for 1 hour and serve. Enjoy!

Stuffed Peaches

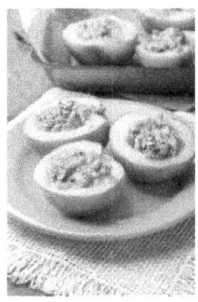

Preparation time: 10 mins

Servings: 4

Nutritional Information: 130 calories, 2g fat, 14g carbs, 10g protein, 18mg sodium.

Ingredients:
- ½ c. favorite dried fruits
- ¼ c. toasted almonds
- 4 peaches
- 2 tbsp. graham crackers
- ¼ tsp. allspice
- 2 tbsp. stevia
- ½ c. fat-free yogurt
- **12 oz. canned peach nectar**

Directions:
1. Scoop each peach, chop the pulp, put into a bowl, add dried fruits and mix.

2. Also add almonds, crackers, sugar and allspice and stir everything.
3. Stuff each peach with this mix, place them on a baking sheet, drizzle the nectar all over, introduce in the oven at 350 degrees F and bake for 40 minutes.
4. **Divide peaches on plates, drizzle pan juices, top with yogurt and serve. Enjoy!**

Dash Diet Doughnuts

Preparation time: 10 mins

Servings: 8

Nutritional Information: 200 calories, 4g fat, 26g carbs, 12g protein, 320mg sodium

Ingredients:
- 3 tbsp. stevia
- 1 c. whole wheat flour
- 1 tsp. baking powder
- 2 tbsp. matcha powder
- ½ tsp. vanilla extract
- ½ c. low-fat buttermilk
- 1 egg
- 1 tbsp. avocado oil
- **cooking spray**

Directions:
1. In a bowl, mix flour with matcha powder, stevia and baking powder and whisk.
2. Add buttermilk, vanilla extract, egg and oil and stir using your mixer.
3. Divide into doughnut cavities after you've sprayed with cooking oil, introduce in the oven at 400 degrees F and bake for 10 minutes.
4. Serve them cold.
5. **Enjoy!**

Berries And Orange Sauce

Preparation time: 10 mins

Servings: 4

Nutritional Information: 100 calories, 2g fat, 20g carbs, 4g protein, 0mg sodium

Ingredients:
- 1 c. orange juice
- 1½ tbsp. stevia
- 1½ tbsp. champagne vinegar
- 1 tbsp. olive oil
- 1 lb. strawberries, halved
- 1½ c. blueberries
- 1 chopped peach
- **¼ c. basil leaves**

Directions:
1. In a pot, mix orange juice with stevia and vinegar, stir, bring to a boil over medium-high heat, simmer for 15 minutes, add oil, stir, take off heat and leave aside for a couple of minutes.
2. **In a bowl, mix blueberries with strawberries and peach wedges, add orange vinaigrettes, toss to coat, sprinkle basil on top and serve! Enjoy!**

Grapefruit Granita

Preparation time: 20 minutes

Servings: 3

Nutritional Information: 80 calories, 0g fat, 14g carbs, 3g protein, 11mg sodium

Ingredients:
- 1 c. water
- 1 c. coconut sugar
- ½ c. chopped mint
- **64 oz. red grapefruit juice**

Directions:
1. Put the water in a pan, bring to a boil over medium heat, add sugar, stir until it dissolves, take off heat, add mint, stir, cover and leave aside for 5 minutes
2. **Strain into a container, add grapefruit juice, stir, cover and freeze for 4 hours before serving. Enjoy!**

Stewed Plums

Preparation time: 10 mins

Servings: 4

Nutritional Information: 110 calories, 2g fat, 12g carbs, 6g protein, 0mg sodium

Ingredients:
- 16 plums
- 1 c. water
- ½ c. coconut sugar
- **5 crushed cardamom pods**

Directions:
1. Put water in a pot, add sugar, heat up over medium-low heat, add cardamom, bring to a boil and simmer for 10 minutes.
2. Add plums, stir gently, cover pot and cook for 5 minutes.
3. **Leave plums aside to cool down before serving. Enjoy!**

Whole Wheat Pumpkin Pancakes

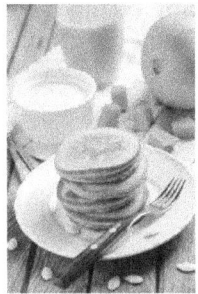

Preparation time: 15 mins

Servings: 8

Nutritional Information: 346 Calories, 14g Protein, 34g Carbs, 19g Fat, 274mg sodium

Ingredients:
- 2½ c. pastry flour
- 2 tbsp. baking powder
- 2 tsp. ground ginger
- 3 tsp. cinnamon
- ¼ tsp. ground cloves
- ¼ tsp. Nutmeg
- 2 eggs
- 2 c. buttermilk
- 1 c. pumpkin puree
- **¼ c, olive oil**

Directions:
1. Combine in a large mixing bowl, flour, nutmeg, baking powder, ginger, cinnamon, salt, and cloves.
2. In a second bowl, whisk together, pumpkin puree, eggs, buttermilk and olive oil. Add wet ingredients in second bowl to dry ingredients in the first bowl.

3. Mix until all is incorporated.
4. Grease and heat griddle over medium flame.
5. Use a quarter cup measure to pour batter and let cook until small bubbles form and the sides set.
6. **Flip and continue cooking until golden brown.**

Pineapple Bowls

Preparation time: 10 mins

Servings: 6

Nutritional Information: 130 calories, 6g fat, 12g carbs, 6g protein, 4mg sodium

Ingredients:
- 4 c. pineapple pieces
- 2 tbsp. honey
- ½ c. whole wheat and barley cereals
- 12 oz. low-fat vanilla yogurt
- **¼ c. coconut, toasted and shredded**

Directions:
1. Divide pineapple pieces into 6 bowls, add yogurt and toss
2. **Sprinkle cereals and toasted coconut on top and serve right away. Enjoy!**

Tofu Chocolate Cake

Preparation time: 10 mins

Servings: 16

Nutritional Information: 190 calories, 35.8g carbs, 2.9g protein, 4.0g fat, 267mg sodium

Ingredients:
- ¼ c. water
- 300 g block of soft dessert tofu
- **One box of super moist chocolate cake mix**

Directions:
3. Preheat the oven to 400 degrees Fahrenheit.
4. Using a blender, blend the tofu and the cake mix together.
5. Once these two have been sufficiently blended, add the water and blend again until smooth.
6. Take the mixture and pour it into a baking dish. This mixture can also make cupcakes.
7. Cook the mixture to the specifications of chocolate cake mix box.
8. **Let the cake cool before serving.**

Chocolate Mousse

Preparation time: 5 mins

Servings: 2

Nutritional Information: 40 Calories, 1g Protein, 3g Carbs, 3g Fat, 76mg sodium

Ingredients:
- ¼ c. unsweetened dark chocolate
- 1¾ c. heavy whipping cream
- ½ tsp. orange extract
- ¼ c. cinnamon
- ½ c. whip cream
- **¼ c. dark unsweetened chocolate**

Directions:
1. Place all ingredients in a blender.
2. Process until desired consistency is reached.
3. **Chill, and top with whip cream and shaved chocolate before serving.**

Conclusion

Congratulations on choosing the first step to fighting hypertension, and weight loss. From this cookbook, the journey will continue to get easier with each day you complete. We hope we were able to set you on the right path in this journey and that you have a good time with all the recipes outlined in the DASH Diet cookbook.

So, the next step is to work hard, dedicate yourself and be determined to ensure that you achieve your set goals by trying to balance your blood pressure and weight loss. The bonus now lies in you. All the suggestions, tips, recipes, and tools all are included in this cookbook. Transform to a happier and better living.

A great thanks for giving us the opportunity to take you through on the DASH Diet journey. Feel free to leave a kind review if you like what you read.

Thank you for purchasing this book. Throughout the course, you must have found out how effective and healthy the diet is. All the recipes incorporated this cookbook have nutrients that help in keeping our bodies fit. The ingredients aids in improving the metabolism and production of enough energy to keep you going.

Kindly consult your physician before you start the diet because its main aim is to reduce blood pressure. Check your blood pressure regularly to keep yourself on the right track.

Happy Dieting!

www.ingramcontent.com/pod-product-compliance
Lightning Source LLC
Chambersburg PA
CBHW071440070526
44578CB00001B/155